A Cardiologist Explains Things

Basic Information for the Layperson

Paul R. Lurie M.D.

and Andrea R. Lurie

Illustrations by Ruben J. Acherman MD

i

DEDICATION

TO LIFETIME LEARNING

CONTENTS

ACKNOWLEDGMENTS

The authors wish to thank the volunteers of Lifetime Learning Institute at State University of New York, New Paltz for providing us the opportunity to present this information in a course to an attentive group of our senior colleagues.. The generous reception of that course led to our conception of this book. We also wish to thank William N. Evans M.D. and his colleagues at Children's Heart Center of Las Vegas NV for permitting the use of many illustrations from their book, "Simple and Easy Pediatric Cardiology." Dr. Evans has also read the manuscript and offered helpful suggestions.. We thank Anne and Ray Smith of Woodland Pond for their invaluable help in final formatting of the book. Carol O'Biso's help with the cover format is much appreciated. Finally, we are in debt to our friend, talented medical illustrator and fellow pediatric cardiologist, Ruben Acherman M.D. for hours of work on the superb illustrations

1

FIRST VISIT TO A CARDIOLOGIST

When you visit a cardiologist or internist for the first time, you have a right to be scared that he or she is going to find something bad about your heart that you were unaware of. Or that he will not give you a chance to tell him about something that is very important to you. Or finally that you will end up getting more information than you can assimilate.

There are a couple of helpful suggestions I would make that you may already know about. Have a relative or friend go with you and sit in the room with you as an observer and if necessary, note taker.

Make a list or even jot down a whole statement that gives the doctor the flavor of your story that he might not get by questioning you. Be sure to give it to him.

You probably are wondering what is the doctor thinking as the encounter begins. I can give a pretty good guess. "Another interesting patient! Can I get the full story out of him and can I solve his problems?"

The interview is structured as is the physical exam that follows. But often, as the doctor finds things on the physical exam he will go back and ask questions about the findings that add substance to the history.

The chief complaint and present illness are the most important part of the history and since we are talking about cardiac problems, they are going to center around one or more of the major cardiac symptoms that are listed here

Breathlessness

Pain
Swelling
Cough
Fatigue
Palpitations (Sense of Abnormal Rhythm)

After that comes past history, family history and social history. As to the latter, he wants to get to know you and as much about you as a person as he can get in a few minutes, but he expects that he will have future opportunities to get to know you better.

Now to the physical examination: This starts with general

appearance, posture, in what position is the patient comfortable, color of skin, other skin problems, nutrition. Next, eye, ear, nose and throat. He looks at the vessels in the retina with the opthalmoscope for clues as to the state of your small vessels. He observes the color of the mucosae, and the state of oral hygiene. He feels the neck for thyroid swelling or nodules or lymph gland enlargement. He listens to the lungs with his stethoscope for normal breath sounds or crackling noises on inspiration called rales, especially at the bases, that signify congestive heart failure.

Exam of the heart itself starts with inspection of the veins in the neck to see at what level of recumbency they collapse. He feels for the edge of the liver and spleen as they descend while you inhale deeply. He presses the skin with one of his fingers just above the ankle to see if a pit forms, signifying edema, the abnormal increase of extracellular fluid in dependent parts of the body. If the history is of a congenital problem, he looks for blueness, cyanosis, and clubbing signifying admixture of unoxygenated blood in the arterial side of the circulation. He feels the pulses in the neck, the wrists, the groin, and the top of the foot. He observes the chest for deformity resulting from chronic overactivity of part of the heart and feels if there is any abnormal lift or heave over the heart. He percusses the heart for abnormal position and size, though he will later have more accurate information on this. Then he listens to the heart with the stethoscope to assess rate and rhythm, the heart sounds and murmurs if any, their location, timing and quality.

He then decides what laboratory tests he wants, most often a chest xray and electrocardiogram, serum electrolytes, creatinine for kidney function, and hemoglobin. Beyond this, he may want an echocardiogram, a 24 hour electrocardiogram recording, or even a stress test. More intensive tests may be needed, either urgently or deferred, depending on his findings.

As I have enumerated his actions here, they sound structured and time-consuming. In experienced hands, however, the structure goes by so rapidly that you are hardly aware of it, and much is accomplished in a few minutes. Unfortunately, today the practice of medicine in the USA does not usually permit the leisurely establishment of a warm personal relationship on one visit.

2

BREATHLESSNESS

In 1915, there were only a few physicians in New York City who called themselves cardiologists. They started an "Association for the Prevention and Relief of Heart Disease." They later changed the name to New York Heart Association, which later became the nucleus for starting the American Heart Association. In 1925, they published this classification (Fig. 2.1) which is still in use today.

Class	Patient Symptoms
Class I (Mild)	No limitations of physical activity. Ordinary physical activity does not cause undue fatigue, palpitation, or dyspnea (shortness of breath).
Class II (Mild)	Slight limitation of physical activity. Comfortable at rest, but ordinary physical activity results in fatigue, palpitation, or dyspnea.
Class III (Moderate)	Marked limitation of physical activity. Comfortable at rest, but less than ordinary activity causes fatigue, palpitation, or dyspnea.
Class IV (Severe)	Unable to carry out any physical activity without discomfort. Symptoms of cardiac insufficiency at rest. If any physical activity is undertaken, discomfort is increased.

Fig.2.1 NYHA Classification - The Stages of Heart Failure. A functional classification that relates symptoms to everyday activities and the patient's quality of life.

You will note that the endpoint of each level is breathlessness. Pain is not mentioned and I will talk a lot about pain in a later chapter. But here, the focus is on shortness of breath, dyspnea.

I became especially aware of the direct effect of an inefficient pump on breathing a few years ago. I was living in an old row house in Albany. We used all three floors connected by two flights of stairs. I ran up and down these stairs many times each day never stopping or slowing down to get my breath. Then one day, in the middle of the second flight up, I suddenly had to stop because of extreme shortness of breath. I took my pulse and found it to be fast and irregular. I had gone from regular rhythm to atrial fibrillation, the commonest abnormal rhythm in old people, and my atrium has never stopped fibrillating. Because the atrium no longer does its duty of filling the ventricle with each beat, it makes the heart as a pump much less efficient. We will discuss abnormal rhythms fully in a later chapter, but here we are going to explore breathlessness.

To really understand breathlessness, we have to consider how the food we eat and the air we breathe together give us the energy to perform work. We will go through several seemingly unrelated but interesting areas to get there:

A cell
Circulation
Muscle structure

How energy is produced without heat
Muscle function
Automaticity of breathing

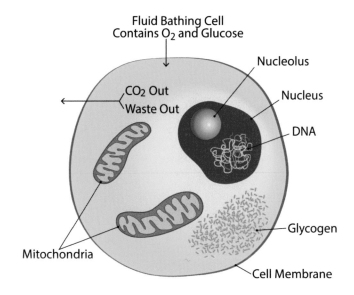

Fig. 2.2 A simplified cell.

This diagram shows only the parts that are relevant to this discussion. Each cell is bathed in extracellular (also called "interstitial") fluid. Think of sea water, the saline fluid that bathed the single-cell primitive organisms from which all life has evolved. Or think back to each of our lives when for a moment we were a single fertilized egg in a saline bath in the mother's uterus. This saline bath contains oxygen and food (glucose) in solution, which enter the cell through its membrane. In turn carbon dioxide and waste products of food used by the cell pass outward through the membrane. In complex organisms with a circulatory system, the extracellular fluid is maintained by the capillary bed that is in intimate contact with every cell. Here it is that the circulatory system meets the cells.

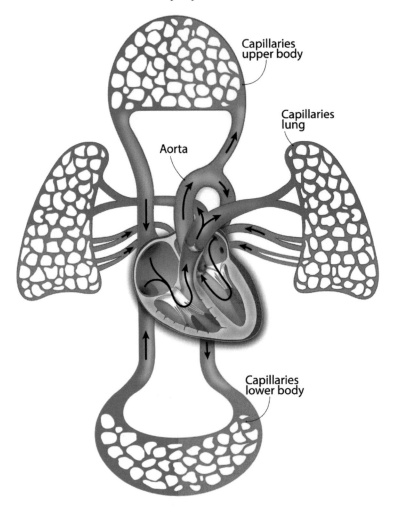

Fig. 2.3 The relation of capillary beds to arteries and veins, both systemic and pulmonary.

This may seem obvious to us today, but it was not understood until 1628 when William Harvey cleared up centuries of confusion by a set of simple experimental manipulations. The diagram of the circulation can be followed around starting with the blue, unoxygenated blood in the two largest veins on the left of the picture with arrows pointing toward the heart. The blood reaches the right side of the heart, (on the left of the picture) where it is pumped into the lungs. In the capillary beds of the two lungs, the blood picks up oxygen and becomes bright red. It then returns to the left side of the heart (on the right of the picture) where it is pumped back out to the arteries that go to the body, eventually branching down to the numerous capillary beds all over the body, where oxygen is released. The blood then becomes dark (blue in the picture) as it is depleted of oxygen and returns via the systemic veins to the right side of the heart.

Figs. 2.4 shows us how a capillary bed can vary its blood flow on demand, as the tiny sphincters, these guardian muscles, contract or relax. The full opening of all these channels in exercising skeletal and cardiac muscles contributes to the phenomenon known as "second wind."

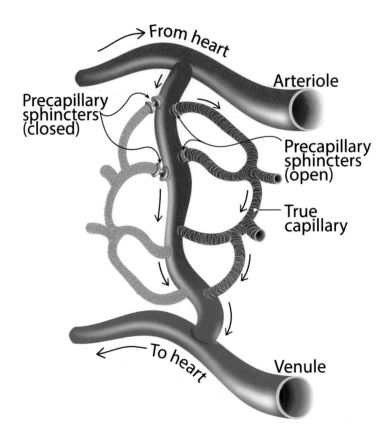

Fig. 2.4 A capillary bed with precapillary sphincters

Returning to the cell, Fig. 2.2, note the nucleus. Here resides the DNA that dictates development, determines with other local factors whether a cell will become bone or brain etc.

The glycogen particles provide instant fuel not dependent on circulation.

Mitochondria are the cellular powerhouse. Every cell that does anything needs these and they are especially well developed in active muscle cells.

This is where food is converted into energy.

Next we turn to the structure of muscle.

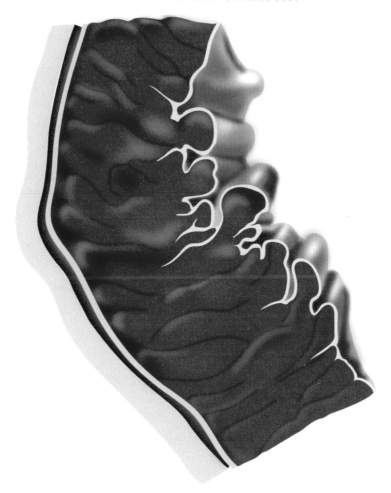

Fig. 2.5. This piece of red meat is a slice of heart muscle magnified .

In most ways heart muscle is similar to skeletal muscle. The main difference is that skeletal muscle needs a nerve stimulus to start it contracting, while heart muscle has its own innate rhythmic stimulation to contract. A slice of heart muscle properly bathed can contract and relax slowly and repeatedly long after its former owner is dead.

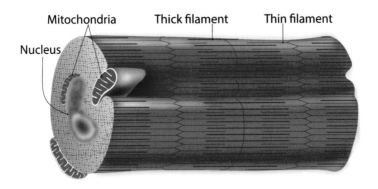

Fig.2.6 With considerable magnification we see an artist's rendition of a part of a single cardiac muscle cell with emphasis on the contractile elements. Also note the nucleus and the mitochondria.

For simplicity we have omitted the capillaries and the transverse tubular system, which aids in contraction and preparation for the next contraction. The arrangement of the bulk of the muscle is better shown by an actual electron microscope picture with much greater magnification, Fig. 2.7, which shows a myriad of fibrils with contrasting stripes. The segment delineated by the arrow is a single unit called a "sarcomere", and it is in millions of units like these that the contractile work of the heart is done.

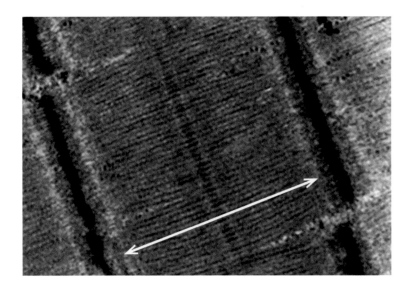

Fig. 2.7. Electron microscopic picture of a sarcomere, the segment delineated by the arrow.

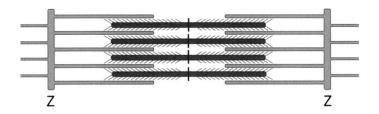

Fig. 2.8. Diagram of a single sarcomere showing the projections from the thick filaments and the overlap of thick and thin filaments which can vary depending on filling of the heart or, in skeletal muscle, the amount the muscle is stretched before contracting.

Before I show you how these segments work, we have to digress for a moment to see just how the energy is produced in the mitochondria so that the segments are enabled to contract.

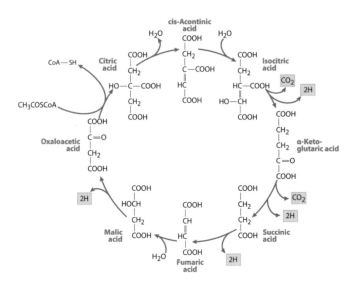

Fig. 2.9 The citric acid cycle

This picture of a chemical cycle that can be bewildering even to a student of biochemistry can be summed up very simply. The food we eat is broken down or converted into glucose which circulates in the blood. In the cell glucose is further broken down into pyruvate which enters this cycle in the mitochondria of any cell in the body that does work. What happens in the cycle is that pyruvate is broken down into simpler and simpler compounds with each reaction using oxygen and yielding a compound with three phosphorus atoms known as ATP, adenosine triphosphate, and carbon dioxide. This compound,

ATP, is the momentary store of electrical energy which it gives up when it is needed for cellular functions by losing one phosphorus and turning into ADP, adenosine diphosphate, a two-phosphorus compound. This is how our body produces energy without producing heat.

Now let us return to the tiny segment of cardiac (or skeletal) muscle and see how, with the energy provided by a supply of ATP, contraction takes place.

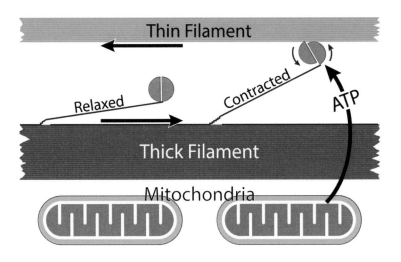

Fig. 2.10 Part of a sarcomere in diagrammatic fashion, to show how a conversion of ATP to ADP supplies energy so that a single arm projecting from the thick filament grabs the thin filament and gives it a yank, then relaxes and falls away. Then another projection repeats the process. These actions are repeated thousands of times with each contraction of the muscle. With each contraction there is a

change in electroyte conditions, most importantly, a release of calcium, and when these conditions change again in a few milliseconds, the contraction ceases.

SARCOMERE

Fully Contracted

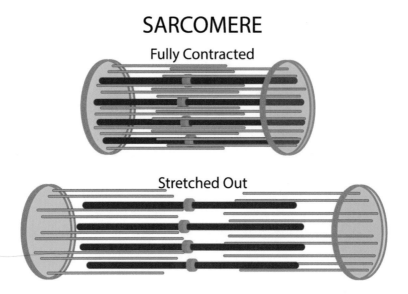

Stretched Out

.Fig. 2.11 A diagram of a single sarcomere of a fully contracted heart muscle and, in contrast a stretched out sarcomere in a heart filled before contraction.

You can see that the strength of a contraction can be varied by the amount of overlap of the thick and thin filaments at the start of a contraction. In the heart, this means that the more the heart is full , the stronger will be the contraction, up to a point. When it is overfull, as in heart failure, there is less overlap so it contracts with less strength.

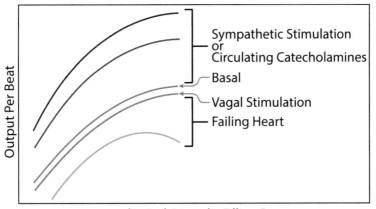

Ventricular End-Diastolic Filling Pressure

Fig, 2.12 Shows how cardiac filling affects strength of contraction and also shows neural and hormonal influences on cardiac contractility. Sympathetic stimulation increases contractility and vagal stimulation reduces it. Catecholamines are mainly hormones from the medulla of the adrenal gland, adrenaline, also called epinephrine. When the heart is failing, unable to keep up with its load, the whole curve shifts to the left so that increasing load results in less effective contraction.

Now that you have a better idea of what is happening in your heart during exertion, you know that the more work the heart and the skeletal muscles do, the more CO_2 is produced. Just how is that related to breathlessness?

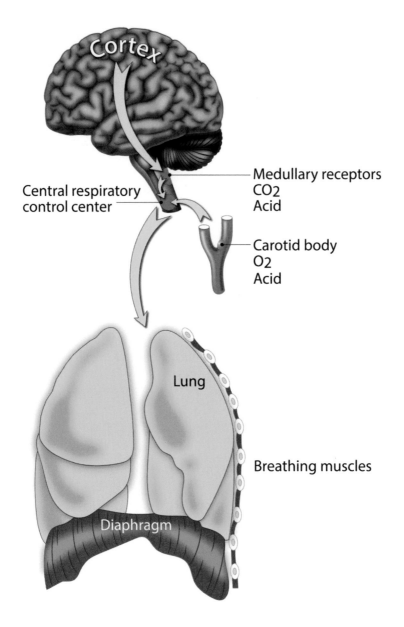

Fig. 2.13 Influence of chemoreceptors on breathing.

The magic word, as in almost every maladjustment that occurs in the body, is RECEPTORS. In the case of CO_2, we have chemoreceptors that are keenly sensitive to acid, (mainly dissolved carbon dioxide) and send stimulating signals to the respiratory center in the brain to get rid of the CO_2. So, as you experience every day, the harder you work, the faster and deeper you breathe. And, if your pump is inefficient or failing, the CO_2 piles up in the blood because it can't be circulated to the lungs and blown away fast enough to keep up with CO_2 production. Thus it becomes obvious that as cardiac efficiency becomes less, the onset of breathlessness is earlier and after less effort. Two of the chemoreceptors concerned with the level of CO_2 are located in the midbrain and the arteries in the neck. Also, you can trace their connection with the respiratory center and its connection with the diaphragm and other muscles that we use for breathing.

Thus we have seen how cardiac and skeletal muscle cells contract and relax using glucose and oxygen and producing carbon dioxide and other wastes, and we now understand that this activity takes place without the generation of heat by the stepwise production of ATP in the mitochondria which allows the storage of energy which is released at the contractile sites in the muscle by conversion of ATP to ADP. The circulation replaces the extracellular fluid bathing the muscles as called for by the acid-sensing chemoreceptors. The strength of cardiac contraction is modulated by intrinsic factors, the degree of stretching in cardiac filling as well as extrinsic factors, both neural and hormonal. We now can understand how the time of onset of shortness of breath is determined by the efficiency of the heart as a pump.

3

THE CIRCULATION AND ITS REGULATION

In this chapter, we are going to look at the circulation as a whole, how blood pressure is produced and regulated and what happens when it gets out of regulation. Let's start with a review of the anatomy of the circulatory system.

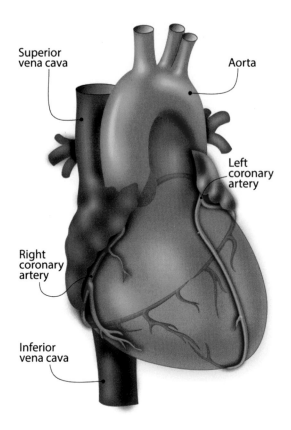

Fig.3.1 The heart from the front.

Note how the coronary arteries emerge from the root of the aorta and some of them are lost to view as they go around to the back of the heart.

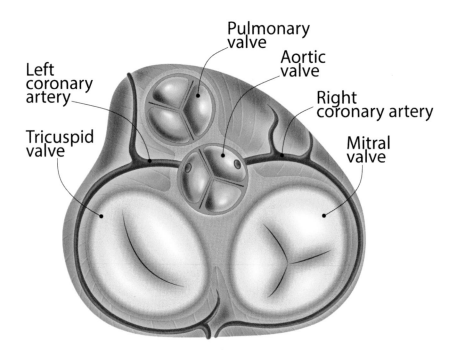

Fig 3.2 Heart from above with atria removed, and aorta and pulmonary artery are transected. In this view the front of the heart is at the top.

This shows the coronary arteries emerging from the aorta just above the aortic valve and their course in the groove between atria and ventricles. This crown-like arrangement gives the name "coronary".

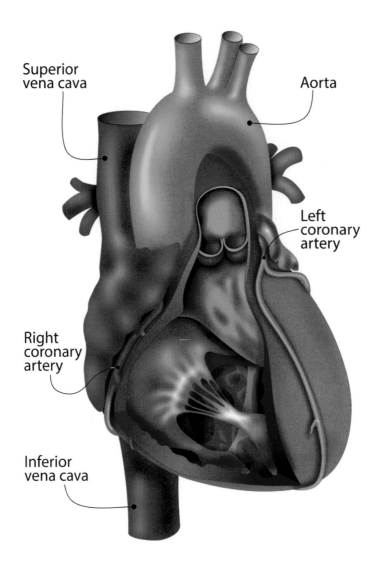

Superior
vena cava

Aorta

Left
coronary
artery

Right
coronary
artery

Inferior
vena cava

Fig. 3.3 The heart opened to the right ventricle with the tricuspid valve leading from the right atrium to the right ventricle and the pulmonic valve from right ventricle to pulmonary artery.

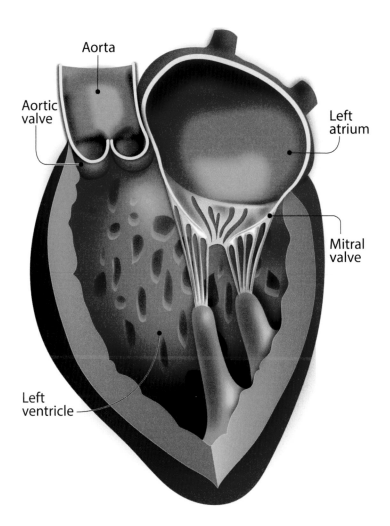

Fig. 3.4 A cut a little farther back shows the left ventricle with the mitral valve leading in from the left atrium and the aortic valve leading out to the aorta.

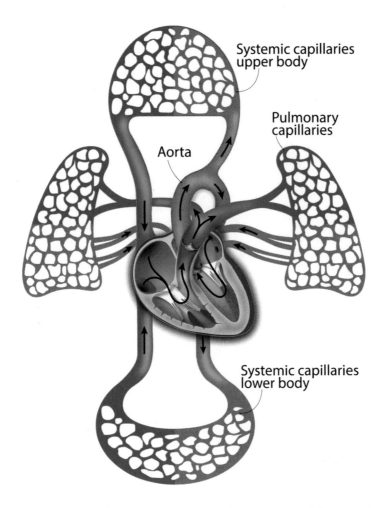

Fig. 3.5 The circulation to show the relation of the capillary beds, both systemic and pulmonary. (Identical with Fig. 2.3)

Again I show you a diagram of the whole circulatory system. Here are the major arteries and veins of the whole system and the capillary beds of both systemic and pulmonary systems. While all of this seems quite simple, I will remind you that for centuries the greatest human minds did not figure out how blood circulated. And Claudius Galen, born 109 C.E., is responsible for that. He was a skillful surgeon who contributed much to medical knowledge. Roman law at the time forbade human dissection, so he studied pigs and primates. Unfortunately, when it came to the heart he was heavily influenced by the current philosophical theories, based mainly on folklore and imaginings. So he fell into and propagated misconceptions which continually were believed, because of his prestige, for well over a thousand years. He professed that what we call the systemic and pulmonary circuits were actually totally separate, connected only by invisible pores in the partition between the ventricles, and that venous blood was continually generated by the liver, and arterial blood was generated by the heart itself. It seems unbelievable that these beliefs lasted until the 1600s when William Harvey, a British physician, got interested in the action of the heart. He studied a wide range of animal subjects, from fish to humans, alive or dead. By careful observation, measurement and experimentation he figured out how blood circulated continuously. He made many demonstrations to colleagues who were hard to convince, and in 1628 wrote a book that devoted many pages to patiently proving the inadequacy of the Galenic concepts and giving solid proof of the concepts we accept today.

Without a microscope he could not say just how the capillary circulation worked. Fifty years after Harvey's death, in 1660, Marcello Malpighi, with one of the first microscopes, described the blood circulating through capillaries in a frog's webbed foot. A typical capillary is just big enough for red cells to squeeze through.

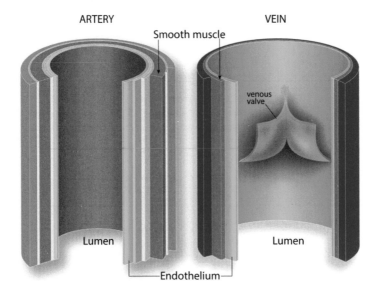

Fig 3.6 Arteries and veins are quite different structurally as shown in this cutaway view. There is much more of both elastic tissue and smooth muscle in the artery wall. The vein has a one-way valve not present in arteries.

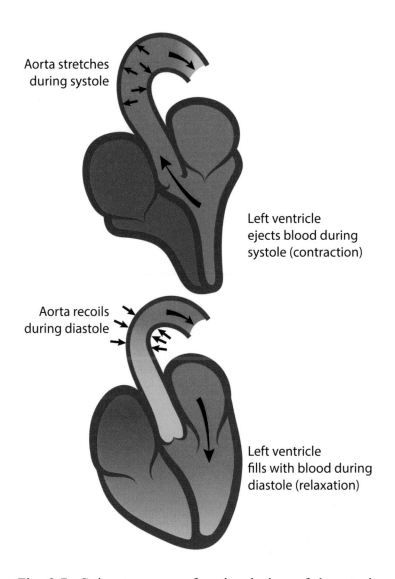

Aorta stretches during systole

Left ventricle ejects blood during systole (contraction)

Aorta recoils during diastole

Left ventricle fills with blood during diastole (relaxation)

Fig. 3.7 Going to a more functional view of the arteries, this figure is very important. It emphasizes the role of all that elastic tissue in the artery wall, which stretches to accommodate the rush of blood in systole (ventricular contraction) and rebounds to maintain pressure and flow during ventricular relaxation, diastole.

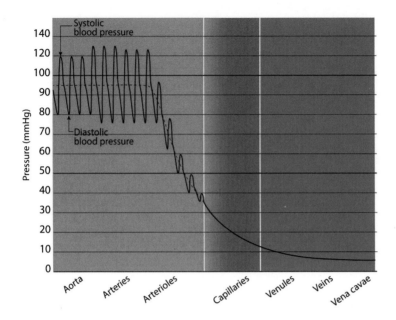

Fig. 3.8 This shows how the full pressure of systole is maintained in the arteries, but falls off in the tiny arterioles. Your radial artery at the wrist is a pretty big artery and its pressure is quite similar to that in the aorta. This is why your pulse at the wrist is a valid indicator of how your heart is pumping. The figure also shows how fully oxygenated bright red blood becomes darker as it releases oxygen in the capillaries.

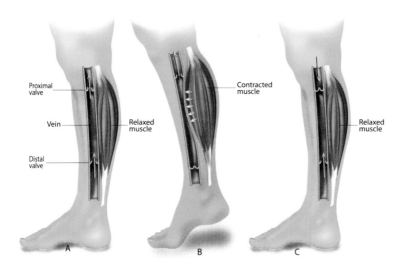

Fig. 3.9 The pressure in the veins is quite low. The flow of blood back to the heart from the legs, though uphill, is maintained by contraction of skeletal muscle around the veins plus the effect of the venous valves as shown. For some veins as we get older, this mechanism fails and we develop varicose veins.

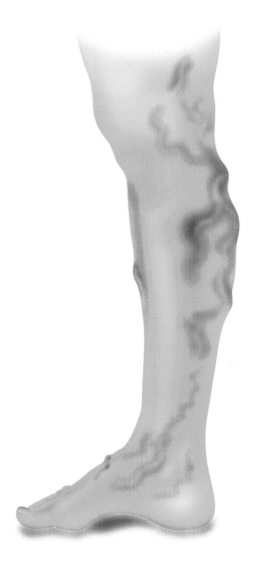

Fig. 3.10 Varicose veins.

This most often happens in superficial veins that do not have skeletal muscle support. The venous valves start to leak backward which dilates the vein and worsens the valve leakage.

Treatment of varicose veins today is most often by heating the vein from the inside with a special catheter. The vein becomes clotted and eventually shrinks into just a ligament-like structure with no blood flow.

Next, it is necessary to consider the way the body is designed to maintain blood pressure within normal limits. We called attention in Chapter 2 to the chemoreceptors involved in breathlessness. Control of blood pressure depends on other receptors. These are called baroreceptors. These receptors are equipped with specialized tissues that are sensitive to stretch. They are located within walls of the aortic arch and the internal carotid artery. They are the start of the reactions that raise blood pressure when it is too low and lowers it when it is too high.

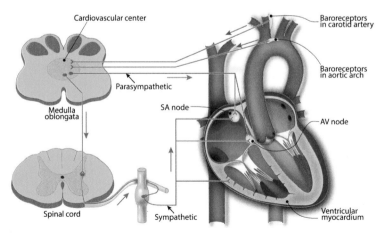

Fig. 3.11 shows the baroreceptors and their sensory

connections with the nervous system. These nerves end in a cardiovascular center in the lower part of the brain. From this center effector or motor nerve connections go out to the various parts of the heart and vascular system. The connections which lower heart rate and contractility pass directly out through the parasympathetic vagus nerves. Other connections pass through the sympathetic system to increase heart rate and contractility and constrict small blood vessels, all of which increase blood pressure.

The nervous system gives us the most immediate control over blood pressure, but, working more slowly over time, there are also hormonal influences as summarized in the following table.

Blood Pressure Regulation by Hormones		
Factor Influencing Blood Pressure	Hormone	Effect on Blood Pressure
Cardiac Output		
Increased heart rate and contractility	Norepinephrine Epinephrine (adrenaline)	Increase
Systemic Vascular Resistance		
Vasoconstriction	Angiotensin II Antidiuretic hormone (vasopressin) Norepinephrine Epinephrine	Increase
Vasodilation	Atrial natriuretic peptide Epinephrine Nitric oxide	Decrease
Blood volume		
Blood volume increase	Aldosterone Antidiuretic hormone	Increase
Blood volume decrease	Aldosterone Antidiuretic hormone	Decrease

Low blood pressure

Now, we will discuss situations where blood pressure is abnormal. First when it is too low, if we are in an upright position, we faint. Fainting is a brief loss of consciousness due to decreased blood flow to the brain. If blood pressure can be obtained during a faint, it is quite low. However, the unconscious period lasts only a minute or two or less and full recovery follows immediately. There is often a brief warning period in which you may feel weak or nauseated and your face may become pale.

There are many causes of fainting. It may be associated with bowel movement, urination, cough or just standing quietly. Sudden emotional disturbances such as seeing a revolting sight or hearing bad news, severe pain, medicines that lower blood pressure, hyperventilation, low blood sugar, excessive bleeding, dehydration, standing up from a recumbent position or sudden onset of a severe cardiac arrhythmia are all possible causes. Some of these are preventable, others not.

To avoid fainting, when possible, guard against dehydration, hyperventilation, and low blood sugar. When prolonged standing is unavoidable, it helps to continue to move the calves in place so as to contract and relax those muscles that massage the veins. Standing from recumbency should be done gradually to allow time for sluggish reflexes to accommodate. If you feel about to faint, find a seat or if none is at hand, squat at once. If you can't do either, at least try to fall as softly as you can.

High blood pressure

The causes of the circulation getting set too high, so that the patient has high blood pressure chronically are most often impossible to figure out.

Thus the term "essential hypertension", meaning we just don't know. The term applies to most cases of hypertension, but we go ahead and treat them regardless. There are a few causes we are able to identify, and here are most of them. Most important are a group of diseases that reduce blood flow to the kidneys, including atherosclerosis, diabetes, polycystic disease, and chronic nephritis.

Among the group that impair blood flow to the kidney: we will be discussing atherosclerosis in detail in a later session; in polycystic kidney, just as its name, many cysts occupy the substance of the kidney and compress the blood supply; diabetes accelerates atherosclerosis; chronic nephritis may result in a shriveled-up kidney with markedly reduced blood supply. All of these raise blood pressure through sensors in the kidney that increase hormones known as the angiotensin-aldosterone system and that causes 1. salt and water retention by the kidneys which increases circulating blood volume as well as 2. generalized constriction of arterioles so that peripheral resistance is raised. Both actions raise blood pressure.

Alcohol: a little may be good. It is a matter under dispute. But over 2 drinks every day or recurring binges have been proven to raise blood pressure chronically. Cold remedies such as Benzedrine, Neosynephrine, or ephedrine are sympathetic-system stimulants and do raise blood pressure. Coarctation of the aorta is a surgically treatable congenital malformation that will be discussed in detail in Chapter 10. It is an hour-glass-like constriction of the aorta where the arch meets the descending portion. It causes hypertension only in the upper body, so it is important that your doctor checks your femoral pulse in the groin when he gets high readings in the arms.

The Valsalva Maneuver

In one degree or another, most of us perform this maneuver a few times a day. It is named after a 17th century Italian scientist who first studied and wrote about it. It describes the sequence of events that follow taking a deep breath and straining against a closed glottis. It can also be produced in a standardized manner by blowing into a blood pressure manometer and keeping it at a fixed pressure for a measured number of seconds. If both blood pressure and pulse are measured simultaneously, initially, there is a slight rise in blood pressure as the heart is compressed. Then, as inflow of blood to the chest is blocked by the high pressure in the lungs, blood pressure falls and heart rate rises. When the strain stops, blood pressure recovers and there is usually an overshoot as it rises above resting value due to reflex constriction of arterioles mediated by baroreceptors and the inflow to the heart of the dammed-up blood in the great veins.. This physiological experiment is duplicated in our daily activities when we strain at bowel movements or lift heavy objects. If we strain too hard or too long, there is the danger that the overshoot may be extremely high and possibly damaging, so it is advisable to avoid long strains and very hard strains.

Drug treatment

When I started in medicine in the 1940s there were no drugs that acted specifically to lower blood pressure. The only treatments were heavy sedatives or surgical sympathectomy, both of which drastically changed one's life. Today's drugs work very well by several different mechanisms, which allows them to be prescribed in combination to get the best effect. I will list them, along with their mode of action:

Diuretics work by reducing the total amount of circulating blood as well as the amount of sodium and water in the vessel walls. Among these are hydrochlorothiazide (Hydrodiuril) and furosemide (Lasix). Spironolactone (Aldactone) is noteworthy as it also has a potassium retaining effect, while the others tend to lose potassium.

Beta-blockers block the effect of adrenaline on the heart and vessels, slowing the heart, lowering cardiac output and lessening peripheral vascular resistance. Examples are carvedilol (Coreg) and propanolol (Inderal).

Calcium channel blockers dilate the arteries and reduce the force of cardiac contractions. Examples: amlodipine (Norvasc) and verapamil (Isoptin).

Angiotensin converting enzyme inhibitors dilate the arteries. Examples: captopril (Capoten) and lisinopril (Prinovil).

Angiotensin II receptor blockers dilate the arteries. Examples: losartan (Cozaar) and candesartan (Atacand).

Salt Intake

The relationship between blood pressure and salt intake has been common knowledge for many years, but it must be emphasized because it is so easily controlled by the individual. Salt (sodium chloride) is an essential component of extracellular (interstitial) fluid. If we ingest more salt than our kidneys eliminate, water is retained, extracellular fluid volume increases and as this includes blood volume, blood pressure rises. Even the extracellular fluid in blood vessel walls increases, stiffening the vessels and increasing their resistance to blood flow and tending to increase blood pressure.

People who have high blood pressure should therefore beware of excessive salt intake. It is not difficult habitually to avoid salty foods, especially snack foods like salty crackers, pretzels and the like. The habit of using the salt shaker before even tasting the food is irrational and can be broken. It is useful to learn gradually to not even put a salt shaker on the table, reserving it for company.

Taking your blood pressure

How best to take your own blood pressure at home? The easiest way to do this, if your doctor requests it, is to invest in one of the automatic machines, so you don't have to learn how to interpret the sounds heard as you deflate the old-fashioned hand-inflated cuff. In any event, you must have a cuff with a bladder that encircles your upper arm and is at least as long as 2/3 the length of the upper arm.

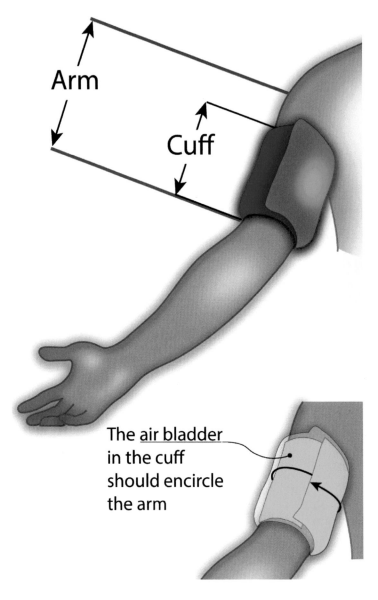

Arm

Cuff

The air bladder in the cuff should encircle the arm

Fig. 3.12 Proper use of blood pressure cuff

If you go for the automatic machine, you should take it in to your doctor's office once a year to have it checked for accuracy. The nice thing about taking your blood pressure at home is that you can avoid the usual tension that attends taking it in the doctor's office, the so-called "white-coat hypertension". Take it while sitting comfortably in a quiet room, usually at the same time and place every time. And be sure to record it for your physician.

4

THE CARDIAC CYCLE

Heart muscle shows a dogged determination to beat, to contract and relax rhythmically. This action leads to several areas of understanding, into each of which I will be giving you a glimpse. There are cardiologists who have spent their whole careers studying heart sounds and murmurs; others have specialized in the electrophysiology of abnormal cardiac rhythms. We will just scratch the surface here, but I feel sure you will find it fascinating.

If you have ever looked through a microscope at the first few cells of a very early egg embryo, you saw that a few of the cells had differentiated into a primitive heart tube that was already visibly beating. That beating would never stop, as long as the hen or rooster it belonged to was alive. Furthermore, if the adult heart were to be excised and put into a saline bath of the correct composition and temperature, it would continue to beat for some hours. Indeed, an excised strip of heart muscle would also contract and relax slowly but rhythmically.

The very name electrocardiogram, tells us that

electricity is involved. The electrocardiogram is a recording from the skin of very low voltages that depolarize the parts of the heart normally in the correct sequence to pump blood efficiently.

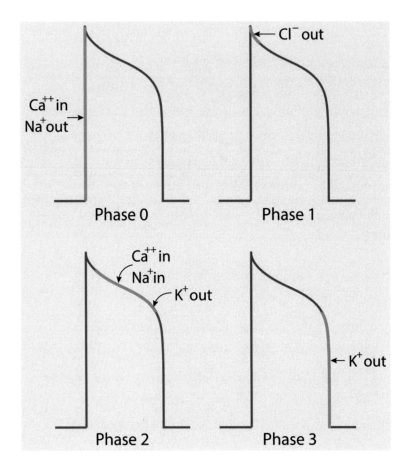

Fig. 4.1 A single cardiac cell's action potentials with associated movements of electrolytes throughout the cardiac cycle.

The changes in the voltage emanating from a single heart cell are associated with important flows of electrically charged chemicals into and out of the cell with each beat. The total of these voltage-changes from all the heart cells reaches the skin to form the ECG.

I am sure you are familiar with today's electrocardiograph machine. Most of us have had a few ECG's, or as many people still call them, EKG's, in homage to Willem Einthoven, the Dutchman who first recorded them as Elektrokardiogramme.

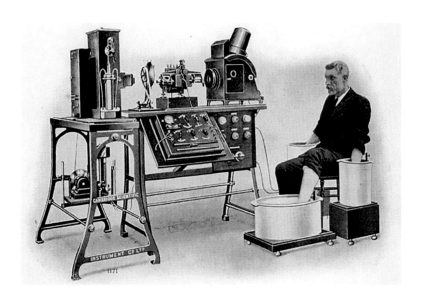

commons.wikimedia.org/wiki/Image

Fig. 4.2 An early EKG.

It was a large table full of sensitive recording equipment. The patient (in this picture it looks like Einthoven himself) sat next to the table with both hands and one foot immersed in pails of salty water. There's quite a contrast between this and the small, compact machine of today, which is even computerized to scan the tracing and produce a diagnostic interpretation. Even today's electrodes are effortless in comparison to the metal plates I used to put on when I started in cardiology in 1948. We had to rub the skin until it was red , then place jelly, then the electrodes.

You may have wondered why the tracing is on squared paper. The answer is standardization. Both the voltage, low as it is, for vertical measurement, and the paper speed for timing of events.

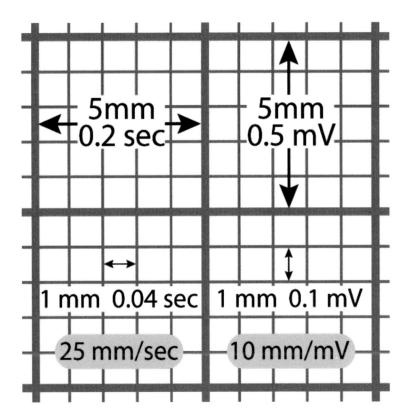

Fig.4.3 Standards for voltage height and paper speed

The usual vertical dimension is 10 mm. = 1 millivolt; and the paper speed is usually 25 mm per second. Thus each small square vertically is 0.1 mv.; and horizontally is .04 seconds.

Any part of the heart with the most rapid intrinsic rate of contraction will take over control of the whole thing. We are going to discuss the process as it occurs with the normal pacemaker in the sinus node located in the right atrium in charge. It may be a bit hard to follow as I am going to put together the electrical impulse that starts in the sinus node, the ECG tracing it makes, the mechanical contraction that follows each stimulus, and the sound the heart makes at each moment.

The sinus node starts a wave of electicity that passes quickly from cell to cell across the atria. That wave of depolarization registers on the electocardiogram as the P wave. It is followed instantly by contraction of both atria which fills the resting ventricles. The electrical impulse reaches the atrioventricular node at the top of the septum between the ventricles, where it is delayed a moment, then the impulse spreads through the ventricles along well defined tracts of specialized conducting tissue.

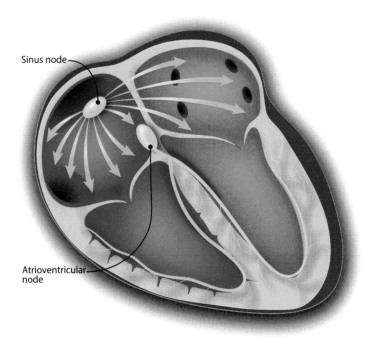

Sinus node

Atrioventricular node

Fig. 4.4 The normal electrical stimulus starts at the sinus node, spreads across the atria, to the atrioventricular node. There specialized conducting fibers spread the impulse across the ventricles.

Depolarization of the ventricles shows on the ECG as the QRS complex, which is followed immediately by the start of ventricular contraction. Ventricular contraction is not as quick and easy as that of the atria. It has to occur in phases. At first it is "isometric", as its muscles and valves tense and pressure builds up until it equals the diastolic pressure in the outflow arteries (aorta for the left ventricle and pulmonary artery for the right). It is this phase that generates the first heart sound.

When pressure is high enough, the valves open and the ejection phase begins. Ejection generates some sounds, murmurs, which we will discuss below. When ejection is finished, the outflow aortic and pulmonic valves snap shut, causing the second heart sound. If either of those valves leak backward, diastolic murmurs are then heard.

Following the QRS, the ECG flattens out for a moment and then shows the T wave of repolarization in preparation for the next beat.

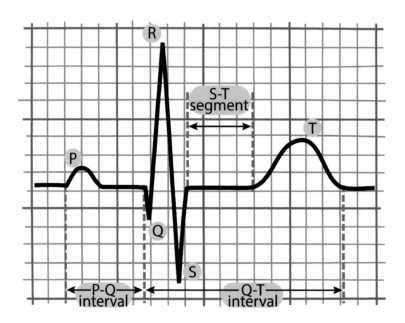

Fig. 4.5 An idealized normal ECG showing well defined P, QRS and T waves.

Heart Murmurs

Murmurs are added sounds, often but not always abnormal, that have more duration than heart sounds. These are named by their timing in the cycle and the anatomical source of the murmur. E.g,, a holosystolic murmur of mitral valve back-leakage is heard throughout systole and is heard best at the apex of the heart, usually the fifth intercostal space in the midclavicular line. An early diastolic murmur of aortic valve back-leakage is heard right after the aortic valve closes and is heard best in the 3rd left intercostal space, close to the sternum. The murmur of pulmonic stenosis, when the valve opens only part way obstructing ejection is simply a systolic ejection murmur heard best along the right side of the upper sternum. Aortic stenosis has similar systolic ejection timing, but is referred higher, into the lower part of the neck. I am not trying to make you into cardiologists and don't expect you to retain this stuff, but am simply emphasizing the basic logic, of both the descriptive words and the acoustic physics underlying them.

There are also commonly heard murmurs that are made by the slight turbulence of normal function. The experienced auscultator recognizes them at once but these "functional" or "innocent" murmurs can cause a lot of anxiety and referrals to consultants, even at times expensive laboratory studies.

Abnormal Cardiac Rhythms

Our next subject, an important one, is abnormalities of cardiac rhythm. First, here is an example of the heart beating too fast, tachycardia.

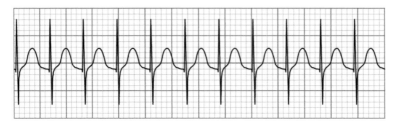

Fig. 4.6 Abnormal tachycardia; there are no P waves.

It is usually quite easy to distinguish such a rhythm from the normal tachycardia of exertion. Normally, a P wave is seen with each beat; abnormal tachycardias usually have no P wave or a small, deformed one. This abnormality can be caused several ways. Usually there is an abnormal residual structure that the electrophysiologist can find using a catheter equipped with numerous closely spaced electrodes. It may be a locus of displaced pacemaker tissue or an abnormal conducting fibrous band. It may occur in bouts of varied lengths or it may be continuous. Occurrences of long duration may lead to the gradual onset of congestive heart failure. There are various medications that can depress that abnormal function and return normal rhythm. If those don't work, an electrophysiologist can pass an electrode catheter into the offending area, locate the abnormal tissue precisely and destroy it, usually by freezing it through the catheter.

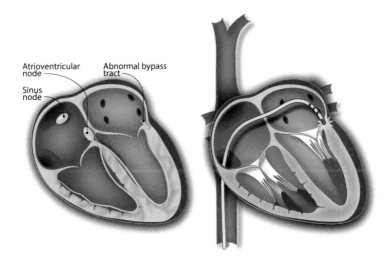

Fig. 4.7 Diagram of one possible source of abnormal tachycardia and its localization and freezing by the electrophysiologist.

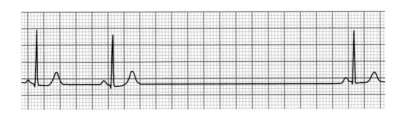

Fig. 4.8 Sinus bradycardia

Bradycardia, excessive slowing, is most often the result of the sinus node losing some of its potency so that it slows down and forgets to put out the next beat. It is called "sinus arrest" or "sick sinus syndrome". Here again, there are medications that help with the problem, but if they don't do the job, the artificial implantable pacemaker can do it.

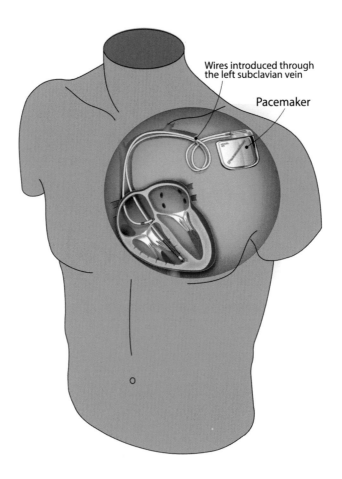

Wires introduced through the left subclavian vein

Pacemaker

Fig. 4.9 The artificial pacemaker is usually implanted under the skin below the left collarbone. Its catheter with sensing and stimulating wires is inserted into the subclavian vein and passed to the right atrium and ventricle.

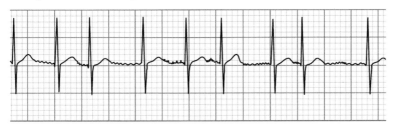

Fig. 4.10 Atrial Fibrillation with absent P waves and fast, irregular ventricular beats.

Atrial fibrillation produces fast, irregular ventricular beats and the ECG shows a wavy baseline instead of distinct P waves. If you were to look at a heart with atrial fibrillation with the chest open, you would see that the atria, instead of contracting rhythmically, are writhing continuously, as if they have totally forgotten that their function is to fill the ventricle before each ventricular beat. This abnormal rhythm is unfortunately one that commonly starts in elderly people who have never had any cardiac problem before. Because of the inefficiency of the heart as a pump that it causes, it is a common cause of exertional dyspnea in the elderly. Treatment with drugs for this is generally either to correct the rhythm, causing the atrium to stop fibrillating and getting sinus rhythm restored; or ignoring the fibrillation, accepting it as inevitable, and reducing the ventricular rate so there is better ventricular filling. It is often possible to stop the fibrillation with a catheter and cold treatment, but this tends to be only a temporary fix for many people.

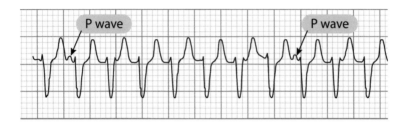

Fig. 4.11 Ventricular Tachycardia

Ventricular tachycardia is the most alarming of all rhythm disturbances because it instantly robs the heart of most of its contractile function and if not successfully treated leads to ventricular fibrillation and death. The treatment for this is electric shock with a defibrillator and if it is diagnosed in time, an implantable defibrillator. You might correctly raise the question, "How did they get this ECG when they should have been trying to attach a defibrillator?" I guess that the patient was under observation with an ECG running when the ventricular tachycardia began.

Some implantable defibrillators permit the preservation of a record that can be retrieved showing the arrhythmia and the time of a discharge of the defibrillator.

When a patient complains of a sensation of abnormal rhythm but when he gets to the cardiologist, his rhythm is back to normal, an electrocardiographic 24 or 48 hour recorder is very useful. It is an accurate way of telling how much of the time the patient's rhythm is abnormal and just what the abnormality is. Today's tiny ECG recorders are very easy to carry around.

Finally, I recommend that anyone interested should learn how to apply and use an external defibrillator. These are now present in most public buildings, hotels, restaurants, and athletic venues and courses are offered to familiarize lay people with their use. In the event that someone suddenly passes out, if their heart has stopped, it may be started back into regular rhythm by the defibrillator. Even if you have not taken a course if you are the only one where a defibrillator is at hand, just stay as calm as possible, follow the directions on the defibrillator and you may save a life.

5

CONGESTIVE HEART FAILURE

Let's start by clearing up any confusion there may still be about the difference between heart failure and heart attack. Neither is a term used by a cardiologist in talking with another cardiologist. They are layman's terms. Rather than heart failure, the cardiologist prefers the term "congestive heart failure" which is exact. We are talking about the gradual buildup of fluid in the body when the heart is unable to cope with its load. There are many possible causes. The heart may be overloaded because of high blood pressure, or an obstructed or leaky valve or it is working inefficiently because of a chronic arrhythmia, or because its muscle is defective as a result of infection, genetic muscle disease like dilated cardiomyopathy or because of atherosclerosis blocking the coronary artery blood supply to some of the heart muscle.

Heart attack is the nonspecific lay term for a sudden noticeable drop in cardiac function for any reason. The commonest cause is myocardial infarction (damage to heart muscle due to loss of blood supply) due to a complication of atherosclerosis causing a coronary artery to become acutely blocked. Another important cause is the sudden onset of a severe cardiac arrhythmia. The latter was discussed in Chapter 4 and coronary atherosclerosis will be covered in Chapter 7.

In discussing congestive heart failure, which is predominantly a matter of the regulation of body fluids, we need a little orientation.

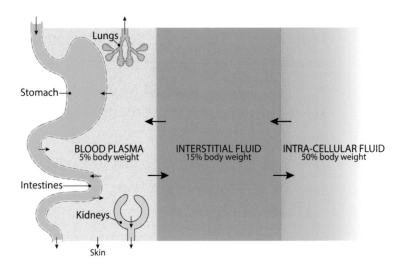

Fig. 5.1 The body's fluid economy. This diagram is helpful. It shows the route by which fluids enter the body through the gastrointestinal system, the different compartments of the body that hold fluid and the percentages of the whole they comprise, and the routes out of the body, the lungs, skin, and kidneys. Note how blood plasma and the fluids around and within the cells of the body interface.

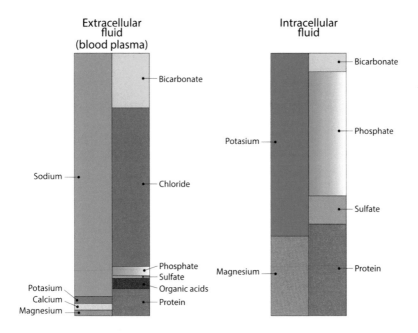

Fig. 5.2 Comparison of the composition of extracellular (interstitial) and intracellular fluid.

The fluid within the cells is nothing like the fluid bathing the cells as shown here. The most important facts are that the major intracellular electrolytes are potassium and phosphate while the major extracellular or interstitial electrolytes are sodium and chloride. The liquid part of circulating blood, that which is not cells or platelets, is called blood plasma. It contains the plasma proteins, albumin and globulin, but otherwise is interchangeable in composition with the rest of extracellular (interstitial) fluid.

As the main function of the kidneys is to stabilize the fluid content of the body, we will now pay close attention to the kidneys. They control the volume and composition of body fluids with the help of hormones, including antidiuretic hormone from the pituitary, the renin-aldosterone system, and natriuretic factors. We will get to these control factors in a bit, but first, let's find out more about the kidneys themselves.

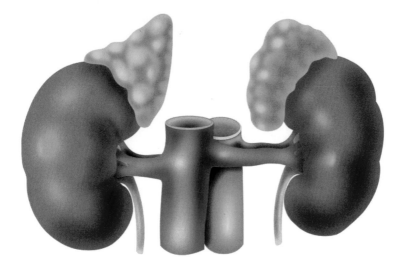

Fig. 5.3 The kidneys with the adrenal glands on top. Notice that the arteries and veins are relatively large, because renal blood flow is large.

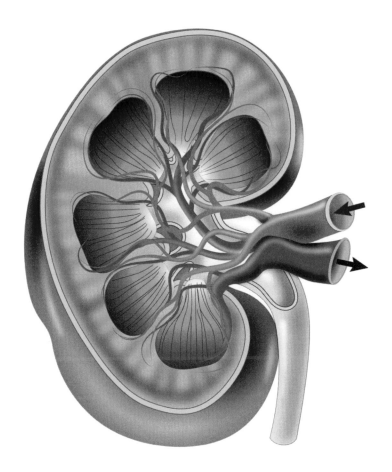

Fig. 5.4 Longitudinal section of a kidney.

This cutaway view shows the arteries and veins and shows the contrast in appearance between the outer cortex and inner medulla. We will see next how the microscopic structure of the kidneys causes this appearance.

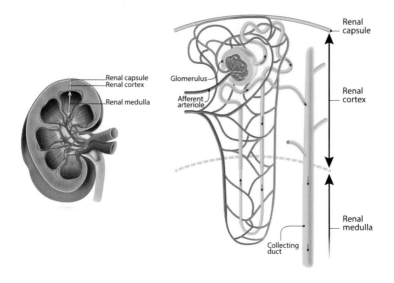

Fig. 5.5 A single kidney unit.

There are about a million of these units in each kidney. It shows how much more vascular the cortex is than the medulla, and the interesting looping structures that make up each unit. Structure is closely related to function. Note the glomerulus, where fluid is filtered out of the arterial blood. In a normal adult, about 200 quarts of fluid filter out of the glomeruli per day, and all but about two quarts are reabsorbed as the fluid passes down the tubules. That two quarts is familiar to us as urine, which passes through collecting ducts into the ureters to the bladder and finally out the urethra.

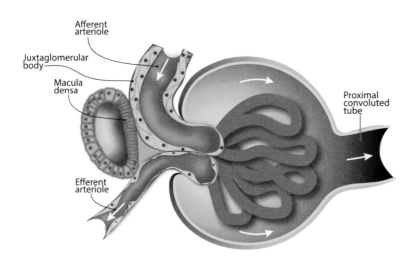

Fig. 5.6 A more detailed picture of a single glomerulus which has been opened up to enable us to see into it.

The glomerulus is designed to filter out large volumes of extracellular fluid from the small arteriole under relatively high pressure. Also note that next to the glomerulus is the juxtaglomerular body, an important organ that helps maintain blood pressure at the proper level. Some of those j-g cells act as baroreceptors so that if incoming pressure is too low, they tell neighboring cells in the j-g body to produce more renin, an enzyme which is the primary trigger of a complex blood pressure regulating system known as the renin-angiotensin-aldosterone system. And to complicate the j-g function even more, note the so-called macula densa cells in the adjacent tubule. These cells are specialized to gauge sodium ion concentration and regulate it by signaling the renin producing cells.

We will come back to the kidney tubule in a few minutes when we discuss diuretics. Right now, to understand better just how edema collects in congestive heart failure, we will return to the interface between the circulating blood and interstitial or extracellular fluid.

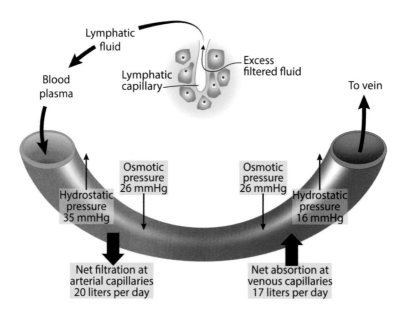

Fig. 5.7 Capillary exchange

This picture takes a lot of explanation, but it is very important in understanding where all the water goes when the heart fails and body weight goes up, and the feet and lower legs swell. If you press the swollen tissue with your finger, a pit forms where your finger was. That is what we call pitting edema. The diagram is of a single capillary.

It shows that at the arterial side of the capillary there is filtration of fluid out of the capillary into the interstitial space and absorption back into the capillary at its venous end. Here is how it happens: At the arterial side, there is an excess of hydrostatic pressure transmitted from the arterial pressure forcing the outward filtration of water, sodium and glucose. At the venous side, the osmotic pressure of the blood pulls water, sodium and glucose back in. There is a net difference; in the diagram, which gives figures for the whole body, it is 20 liters per day out, 17 liters per day reabsorbed. The difference is absorbed by the lymphatic circulation, which ultimately gets back into the veins, but slowly. If central pressure in the veins rises due to congestive heart failure, this will retard lymphatic reabsorption as well as reabsorption into the venous side of the capillary bed. Thus you can see how interstitial fluid volume increases with congestive failure. It also explains how more fluid collects in dependent parts of the body, as the hydrostatic pressure is higher there. When edema forms in the lungs, it forces one to sleep in a semi-sitting position with several pillows. This moves the fluid out of the upper part of the lungs, so there is at least some lung available for gas exchange.

Congestive heart failure is treated by several

routes, usually at the same time. The quickest results are obtained with diuretics and there are several different classes, according to the part of the kidney that they affect.

The most frequently prescribed and probably the most effective diuretic is Lasix (furosemide). It is in the class of "loop diuretics" because it works in the part of the tubule with the sharp reversal known as the loop of Henle. The thiazide diuretics work near the next bend in the tubule and the potassium sparing diuretics, most notably Aldactone (spironolactone), work still farther down, just before the collecting tubule empties into the renal calyx and the start of the ureters.

What all diuretics do is reduce the amount of reabsorption of fluid as it goes down the tubules. The physician supervising a patient on diuretics is concerned with his serum electrolytes, especially potassium, which may be at times excreted in excess, leading to abnormal muscle function. He usually recommends frequently eating bananas, as they are an excellent source of potassium, but there are many other sources.

At the same time, the physician prescribes various drugs that decrease the peripheral resistance against which the heart has to pump. These drugs work by different modes of action but all produce the same effect, namely they dilate small arterioles. Most of them also cut down on the work of the heart by slowing heart rate. Because of these actions, many of the drugs that treat congestive heart failure are the same or close relatives of those that treat hypertension: beta blockers, calcium channel blockers, ACE inhibitors, and angiotensin II receptor blockers.

Next, I'll say a word about what happens when the kidneys fail completely. There are now a couple of effective ways to manage this. The first is a trip to a dialysis center 3 times a week and staying hooked up to an artificial kidney machine for about 3 hours each time.

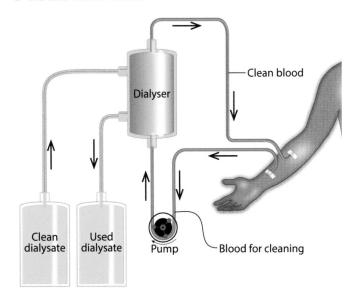

Fig. 5.8 The artificial kidney.

This diagram gives you an idea of how those machines function. Usually a loop is surgically created between an artery and a vein in an arm. This is filled with an anticogulant and locked until dialysis starts when it is opened to the machine. Blood from the artery goes into the machine and returns from the machine to the vein. In the dialyzer itself, a membrane separates the blood from a saline bath into which the waste products diffuse.

The other method of managing renal failure is kidney transplant, which is not easy to get, but very effective.

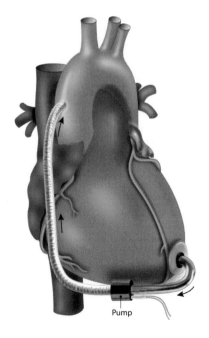

Pump

Fig. 5.9 Left ventricle assist device

Finally, you all know that if the heart fails completely, a few lucky people can get cardiac transplants. But you may not be aware that there have been some remarkable technical improvements in mechanical hearts that can help the failing heart for increasing lengths of time, some going successfully for several years. The type shown in Fig. 5.9 is one that has a high speed cylindrical motor without bearings that impels blood constantly from left ventricle to aorta without any sense of pulsation. It is powered by an implanted battery which can be charged through the skin by induction. And on that optimistic note, I will quit the subject of congestive heart failure.

6

HEART-LUNG INTERRELATIONS

First, a little pulmonary anatomy. The lungs are very soft and spongy, built for their function of exchanging gases with the air we breathe. For a review of the circulation of unoxygenated blood from the right ventricle and pulmonary artery into the pulmonary capillary bed then returning via the pulmonary veins to the left side of the heart, bright red and loaded with oxygen, you are referred again to Fig. 2.3.

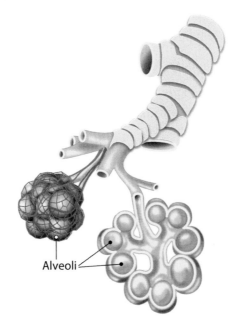

Fig. 6.1 Pulmonary alveoli.

This picture shows you the end of the line in the bronchial tree, two alveoli, one open so you can see the inside of the air sac where the gas exchange takes place.

Normally, the right ventricle pumps as much blood into the pulmonary artery as the left ventricle pumps into the aorta with each beat. As the lungs are spongy structures and are in very close contact with the heart it is not surprising that pulmonary peripheral resistance and pulmonary artery pressure are quite low in comparison to those on the systemic side. In fact systolic pressure in the pulmonary artery is normally around 25 mm of mercury, while that in the aorta is about 125.

As you will recall from discussion of congestive heart failure in the previous chapter, when the heart cannot expel its load fully for any reason, pressure builds up behind the part that is failing. To take an example that is very localized, mitral stenosis, a nearly closed mitral valve, scarred by previous rheumatic fever. This used to be very common in the days before penicillin, and is still common in developing countries. The result of this blocked valve is a rise in pressure in the left atrium. That is reflected directly in the pulmonary circuit as the pulmonary venous pressure rises, leading to a rise in the pressure in the pulmonary capillaries, the pulmonary artery, and the right ventricle. To summarize, anything that causes failure of the left side of the heart will be reflected in a rise in pressure in the pulmonary circuit. This can result in edema of the lungs with cough, sometimes bloody sputum, breathlessness and even at times bronchospasm with wheezing suggesting an asthmatic attack. When the doctor with stethoscope asks you to take a deep breath, he is listening for crackling noises called rales, that are an early sign of pulmonary edema.

As you already know, there are many problems in the heart that can cause congestive failure. These include damage from coronary artery blockage, various heart muscle diseases, cardiac arrhythmias, hypertension, other valve problems causing either forward obstruction or backward leakage, and various congenital malformations. Any of these can cause the pressure to back up in the lungs.

But we also have to consider the effect of diseases of the lungs themselves and how they affect heart function. While there are whole books devoted to this subject, it can be summed up fairly simply if you understand some facts, namely that any lung disease if severe enough, may disturb gas exchange, raise the level of carbon dioxide and lower the level of oxygen in the lungs and the circulating blood. The small arteries of the lungs are very sensitive to these changes in oxygen and carbon dioxide and respond by constricting, and if the gas exchange abnormality continues, the arterioles become permanently thickened. Raising the resistance of the whole pulmonary vascular bed increases the pressure in the pulmonary artery, right ventricle, right atrium, the veins of the neck and the liver. This is how we get congestive heart failure resulting from chronic lung disease.

7

SEEING INTO THE HEART

How do physicians see into the heart? We will go historically from the first simple xrays to the most advanced current modes of seeing into the heart.

Xray of the heart. For years this was all there was and we did the best we could with it. With xray, we are just looking at the heart's shadow, NOT seeing into it, but it came first, is easy to get and requires very little labor and equipment that is widely available. This includes both plain films and fluoroscopy and both can be complemented by a swallow of barium which outlines an enlarged left atrium that pushes aside the esophagus.

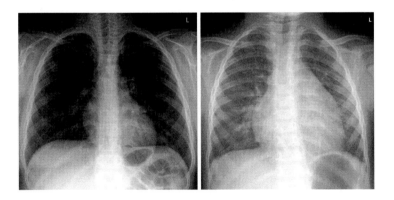

Fig. 7.1 Contrasts a normal chest xray (left) with one that shows pulmonary congestion and cardiac enlargement.

Electrocardiography. We have talked at length earlier about this. It can give us information about the rate and rhythm of the heart, as well as cardiac enlargement and condition of the heart muscle. It is especially good for detecting localized damage to heart muscle due to coronary artery disease. Nowadays, it is quick and easy, painless, harmless, performable by a tyro, while yielding a lot of important information. So, it is still part of what cardiologists do.

Next we will turn our attention to the development of methods that involve injecting xray-opaque materials into the blood stream to photograph a shadow of the inside of the beating heart— angiocardiography. The story starts in Cuba, in 1937. A brilliant pediatrician named Agustin Castellanos wanted to learn more about how the congenitally malformed heart functioned. He knew only that there was available an iodine-containing solution that could mix with blood and show up in blood vessels on xray. He found, first in animal studies, then in humans, that this material, known as diodrast, could be injected harmlessly, except for an intense sensation of heat all over the body that only lasted for a moment. If you timed it right, you could get a picture of the inside of the heart by a single xray exposure when the blood mixed with diodrast went through it. In the years to follow, there were many improvements on his technique in all of its aspects.

Drug companies worked on the contrast substances with gradual improvement until there were no symptoms detected by the patient and minimal disturbance of the osmotic pressure of the blood.

Xray equipment was improved. First there were home made mechanical plate changers coordinated with the triggering of xray exposures. These were replaced with image amplifiers Fig. 7.2 that turned a low intensity fluoroscopic image into a clear, intelligible picture that could be captured on a movie camera as well as observed on a screen at the same time with a 2-way mirror. Later digital recording of the image replaced the movie camera, enabling immediate study of the picture on the computer or TV screen instead of having to develop and project it.

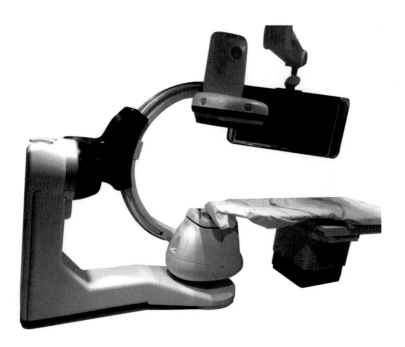

Fig.7.2 A modern image amplifier with digital recording

Instead of injection of the contrast into a peripheral vein, the injection was made into the heart itself as close to the suspected abnormality as possible, through a catheter, first by hand injection, later by mechanical high speed injectors.

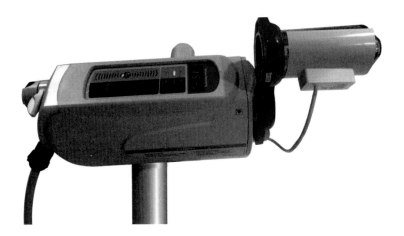

Fig. 7.3 A mechanical injector, showing the heated syringe and connections for high air pressure.

All of these developments took place over the span of many years.

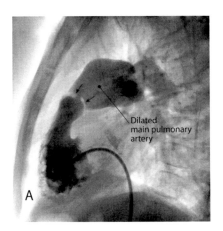

Fig. 7.4 A single frame from angiocardiography of valvar pulmonic stenosis, showing the thickening and doming of the valve and the jet of blood forced through the narrow opening. Arrows point to the valve.

Next, we will talk about how that catheter got into the heart. The development of cardiac catheterization is fascinating. When I sat in a lecture hall at Columbia University College of Physicians and Surgeons in my senior year, in 1942, a few months after Pearl Harbor, I was charmed by a professor with a foreign accent named Andre Cournand (Fig. 7.5) who told us about his findings with heart catheterization. Because of the war, he and his colleague, Dickinson Richards (Fig. 7.6) were working in a basement lab at Bellevue Hospital, studying cardiac output in accident victims in various stages of shock. How do you accurately measure cardiac output in order to evaluate various treatment regimens for shock? The answer is the Fick principle, developed in 1870, that uses three variables, the oxygen used per minute, which can be arrived at by measuring the amount of air expired in a minute and analyzing its gases; the oxygen content of the blood entering the lungs which can be sampled by a catheter passed from a vein into the right side of the heart where a good mixture of all the blood returning from the body is available, and the oxygen content of blood leaving the lungs, sampled through a needle in an artery. Little did I know that Cournand and Richards would later get a Nobel prize for their ground-breaking studies, nor did I have any idea that in a few years I would be running a cardiac catheterization lab myself, not to study shock, but to diagnose congenital heart malformations. All of those technical developments in angiocardiography and cardiac catheterization that I just related were experienced intimately and contributed to by me in the years that I was actively working as a pediatric cardiologist, from 1948 to 1982. But I will get to more details of that in our final session.

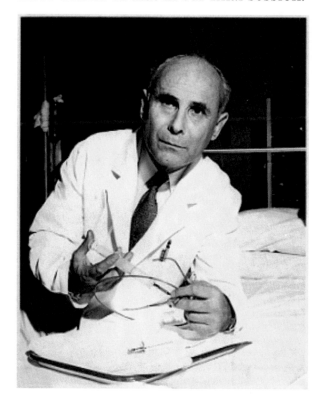

Fig. 7.5 Andre Cournand M.D., with cardiac catheter, c.1956

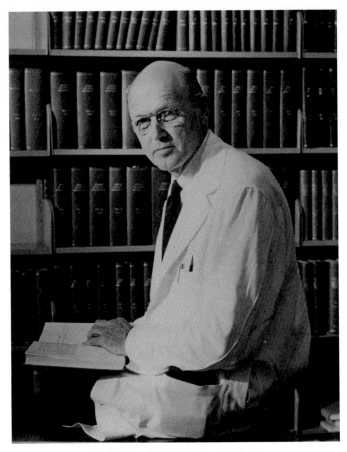

Fig. 7.6. Dickinson Richards M.D. c.1960

Echocardiography. Just as we all were settling back securely in the belief that we were already in the best of all possible worlds, the world caught up with us in the shape of echocardiography. Finally, the clinician is able to actually see into the heart in real time, with the patient located wherever is convenient viz. exam room, bedroom, operating room, emergency room, or admitting room. Now, to most cardiologists, echo is an extension of the elements of the physical examination: inspection, palpation, percussion, and auscultation. In a situation of suspected congestive failure, for instance, instead of looking just for expanded neck veins that don't collapse when they should, feeling for an enlarged liver, listening for rales at the bases of the lungs, etc., with echo, he or she looks directly at a heart that is overfull in systole and diastole, a mitral valve that leaks backward in systole, and a layer of excess fluid in the sac around the heart. What an advance this is!

I still recall in the last few years of my last real job, heading the division of cardiology at Childrens Hospital of Los Angeles, in the late 1970's and early 80's after echocardiography had progressed to the point of clear images in two dimensions, when a new patient came in, he was taken directly to the echo machine, before anyone bothered to take a history or do a physical exam. It made such a difference to the speed at which one could assess the patient's problem (At least the physical part of it). I was very worried that trainees would get into bad habits and the keystones of good medicine would be dismantled before they mastered them (including the social history which is so important in dealing with parents trying to come to grips with the fact that they have a child with a heart problem). Fortunately, my fears were unfounded. Fellows in training still take histories and do physical examinations. But, they go on to the echo almost immediately.

I'd like to go back a bit to some of the history of echocardiography. You probably all know a little about sonar, the method developed in World War 2 to detect submarines, and also to detect depth in shallow waters. It depended on sending out pings of sound and timing their reflections from the bottom, or the hull of a sub. Shortly after the war, a Swedish cardiologist at the University of Lund named Inge Edler was trying to help his surgeon colleague who was reaching into the beating hearts of patients with his finger to break open stuck mitral valves. He thought the sonar principle could be helpful but needed a physicist to work with him. He found a willing helper in a young man named Hellmut Hertz and together they, working with some engineers at the local shipyard, developed what has been called the first ultrasonic cardiograph in 1953. Edler's interest was focused on the mitral valve and he developed some theories based on faulty observations with the result that little attention was paid to his work. However, the two are now given credit for being the first to use ultrasound for cardiac research.

In contrast, an American cardiologist named Harvey Feigenbaum (Fig. 7.7) came along a few years later, ignorant of their work and starting with a primitive echo machine used by neurologists to detect shift of the midline of the brain, did some careful, practical studies that were gradually accepted and opened the door for further engineering advances in ultrasound development. As an interesting sidelight on Dr. Feigenbaum, he was one of the brightest students I had when I taught at Indiana University School of Medicine. He always asked the right questions. I saw him recently in Indianapolis, where he is still actively teaching at age 82 and he related to me an interesting story about how by a couple of coincidences he fell into echocardiography.

He was on the full-time staff of cardiology at Indiana, doing research on methods of measuring the volume of the left ventricle as it contracted and relaxed. He received a junk-mail letter advertising a sonic instrument that could be used to measure ventricular volume. He phoned and was told that they would have the instrument on display at an upcoming cardiology meeting which Harvey planned to attend. When he got to the booth, it was manned by a person who knew only about its neurological use to detect shift in the midline of the brain, nothing at all about cardiology or ventricular volume. But he allowed Harvey to put the transducer over his heart and there on the screen was a dot that moved with his heartbeat. Disappointed but piqued a bit, when he got home, he went to the Neurology Dept. and borrowed their sonic machine. He got a cardiac surgeon to help him in the animal lab. They put a needle in a dog's pericardial sac and injected saline. The single moving dot, which turned out to be the back wall of the heart, immediately became two dots as the heart was separated from the pericardium by fluid and they then reversed the process by removing the fluid. He was able to repeat this finding in more animals and reported it. In the next piece of luck, a couple of other investigators tried to duplicate this but could not because their instruments, made by a different company, were not properly focused. By this time, Harvey knew he had something important and convinced a manufacturer to assign some engineers to give detailed attention to the application of ultrasound to heart disease.

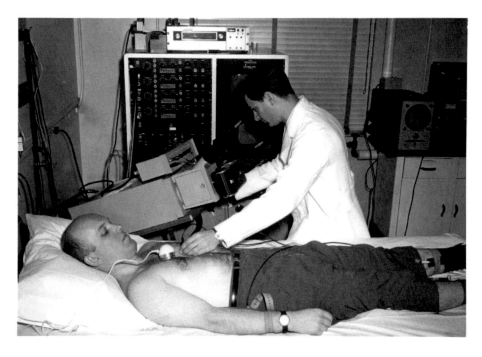

Fig. 7.7 Harvey Feigenbaum performing an echocardiogram, about 1964

As the available equipment gradually improved, he wrote several convincing papers and made more discoveries and by 1972 had enough material to write the first edition of his textbook, "Echocardiography". He even is responsible for that name, which now supersedes other terms such as "cardiac ultrasonography". His book is now in its 7th edition, as new contributions by numerous investigators and advances in technology have come along so rapidly.

The technology involved with getting a beautiful

image of the inside of a beating heart has advanced in ways that were not dreamed of in the early days. These include making echo instruments adjustable in frequency, depth of focus, and other parameters to maximize clarity. What started as sort of an ice pick view that was meaningless to most people suddenly became easily understood when a fan-like view of two dimensions became available. And now three dimensions are possible, though not yet used routinely. Applications of the Doppler effect (the change in frequency of a train whistle as it approaches and recedes) permit measure of blood flow and estimating pressure in localized parts of the heart and there are even methods of studying contraction within the ventricular wall itself. I will demonstrate some of these in a moment, but I must apologize, they will be still pictures, not the beautiful movies that the echocardiographer sees. As advances in echo technology continue to this day, the large machine that Harvey once used is now much more compact, and it is even possible to get a pocket size one for less precise use.

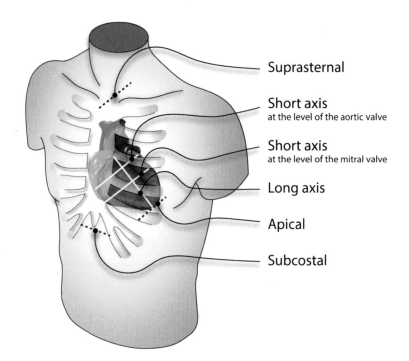

Suprasternal

Short axis
at the level of the aortic valve

Short axis
at the level of the mitral valve

Long axis

Apical

Subcostal

Fig. 7.8 The standard 2 dimensional views of the heart by echo. Each view looks at a fan-shaped section as the lines indicate. This is done by positioning the transducer as shown.

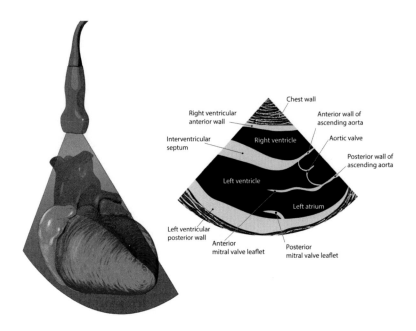

Fig. 7.9 Parasternal long axis view

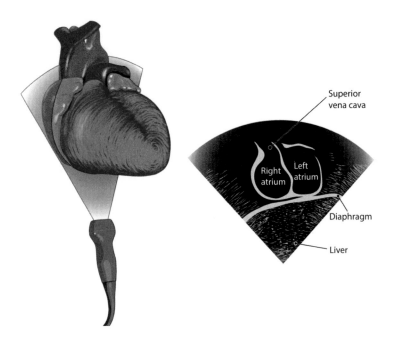

Fig. 7.10 Subcostal view of the atria

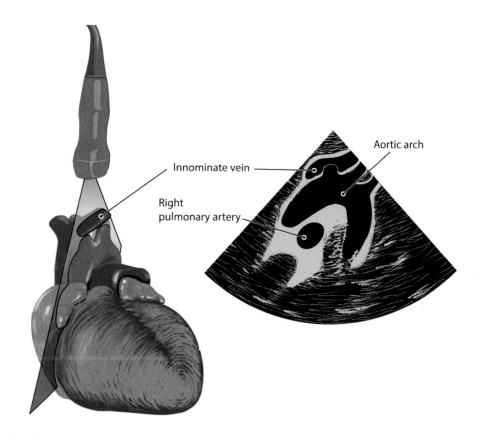

Fig. 7.11 Suprasternal aortic arch view

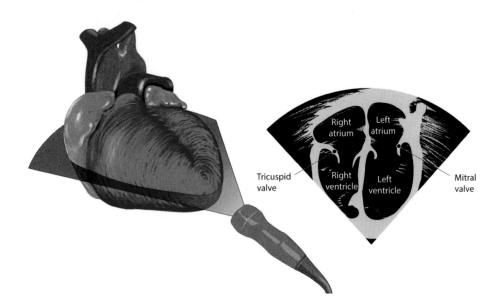

Fig. 7.12 Apical 4 chamber view

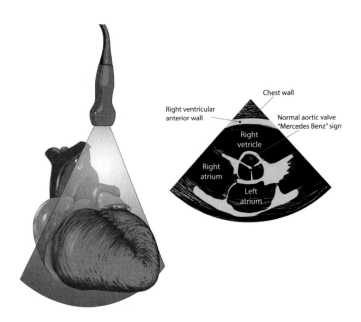

Fig.7.13 Parasternal short axis view at aortic valve level

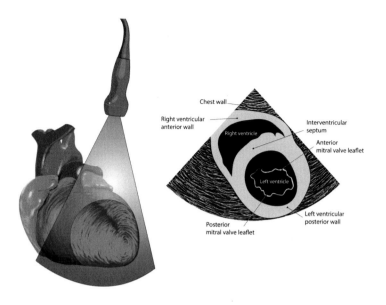

Fig. 7.14 Parasternal short axis view at mitral valve level

I must mention one other application of echo, that is, when the transducer, specially designed for the purpose is sent down the esophagus, most often in an anesthetized patient in the operating room. With this application, an echocardiographer can collaborate with a surgeon to assess immediately, whether the surgeon has accomplished his surgical goal completely.

We have talked at length about echocardiography because it is now completely accepted and of such value that it has replaced most diagnostic catheterizations and contrast angiocardiography. A major exception is coronary arteriography, pictures of the coronary arteries as they emerge from the base of the aorta. A movie made during injection of contrast directly into the origin of each coronary artery shows a detailed road map to be followed by the surgeon or interventional cardiologist. At first, injections were made in the root of the aorta. Mason Sones became a pioneer in this field. Accidentally during an injection into the aortic root, his catheter unintentionally whipped into a coronary artery and gave him a much sharper picture. Finding that it did no harm, he began to do it intentionally and published his findings. (See Fig. 8.2, page 115)

Next, let us turn to cardiac computed tomography (CCT) and cardiac magnetic resonance imaging (MRI). They both can produce detailed 3-D images. They are only used occasionally because of the superior availability of echo. Both require expensive major installations, usually in large hospitals. CT has a further disadvantage of increased xray exposure, but it is quick and yields a lot of information. Both studies require a quiet patient, so some patients, especially young children, may need general anesthesia. As far as is now known, the intense magnetic fields of MRI are harmless. (I have to say from personal experience that the claustrophobia during an MRI study can be close to intolerable.)

How do they work? CT is essentially a circular array of small xray tubes and receivers opposite each. These are discharged in a rapid sequence and a computer does the rest, synthesizing 2D and 3D pictures.

MRI is much more mystifying. The strong magnetic field shakes up the hydrogen atoms in the area of the body being examined and they emit energy which is translated into images.

8

HEART PAIN

In 1915, when the New York Heart Association published its classification of cardiac symptoms, pain is not mentioned. It was all about degrees of breathlessness, which we discussed in Chapter 2. This chapter is about pain. Perhaps the reason it was not part of their classification is the belief at that time that cardiac pain meant certain death. Dr. James B. Herrick changed all that, but it took time. In 1912, he showed from personal study of patients that angina pectoris need not be fatal and a few years later he showed how the electrocardiogram could be used to diagnose and follow the course of coronary thrombosis and occlusion. He showed that it was possible over time to develop collateral circulation to areas of cardiac muscle whose main blood supply was occluded. Eventually, the attitudes of cardiologists changed and we now have much attention focused on the pain associated with diminished blood supply to heart muscle.

At the outset, I must emphasize that anginal pain may be either a recurrent pattern brought on by a certain level of exertion or other stress, and relievable by rest and/or a nitroglycerin tablet under the tongue, or in contrast, the result of an infarction that no simple treatment can alleviate, a real emergency that needs immediate intervention.

The pain may be brought on by exertion, emotion, stress, or even occur in sleep. The typical angina pectoris which translates to "squeezing of the chest" is just that, a painful sense of squeezing in the front of the chest, radiating to the shoulders, arms, neck or jaw.

But there are less obvious symptoms that may be all some people have such as pain in the upper back, nausea, vomiting, profuse sweating, loss of appetite, loss of energy, intense feelings of dread, even shortness of breath (still here, not gone away).

You are now familiar with the anatomy, at least of the major coronaries as they emerge from the aorta just beyond the aortic valve. Take another look at Figs. 3.1 and 3.2, pages 28 and 29, if you would like to review this.

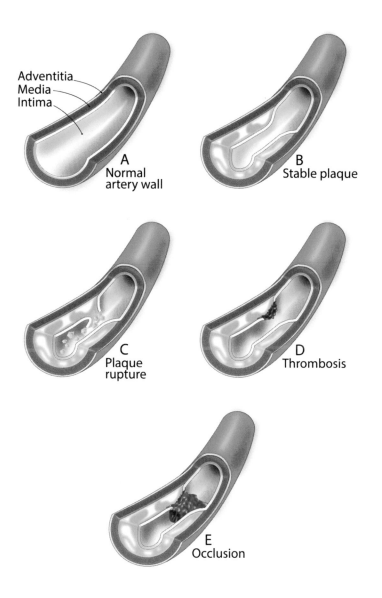

Fig. 8.1 Progression of plaque in an artery as it gradually approaches the point where it occludes an artery.

The rupture of a plaque can lead directly to materials passing down into smaller vessels to cause damage, or to attached clot which occludes the lumen at the plaque site or to clots forming on the plaque and being dislodged into smaller vessels downstream. Keep in mind that an artery does not have to be completely occluded to cause symptoms.

Besides the damage to coronary arteries, similar problems may occur in arteries anywhere in the body, but they cause different problems in different places. In the brain, they cause strokes, in the kidney they cause hypertension. (Remember the juxtaglomerular apparatus!) In arteries of the legs they cause pain on ambulation called by the euphonious term, "intermittent claudication" as well as in more severe cases, gangrene. By weakening the arterial wall atherosclerosis can cause a progressive dilation which we call an aneurysm. (Aneurysm will be discussed later in this chapter.)

What causes a plaque to start forming? It is now considered to be an inflammatory process with various cells invading the inmost layer of the vessel and the body putting forth other cells in a defensive reaction. Soon cholesterol from the circulating blood starts collecting in the growing plaque and makes up a large part of it.

The fact that there is so much cellular activity in the plaque has led to the relatively new concept that it is possible to treat a patient aggressively enough to reduce the size of plaques.

In 1987, Dr. David Blankenhorn of the University of Southern California published the first definitive proof that in patients on successful treatment with statins there was actual regression of plaque. This was a randomized, placebo-controlled study of 162 non-smoking men, age 40 to 59 years with previous bypass surgery. The study ran for 2 years in order to get definitive results.

There follows a list of risk factors associated with worsening of atherosclerotic vascular disease.

Smoking
Diabetes
Obesity
Inactive life style
High blood pressure
High blood LDL (low density, bad) cholesterol
Low blood HDL (high density, good) cholesterol
High blood triglycerides
Stress

Activity. In 1953, Dr. Jeremy Morris studied 31,000 London Transport workers. He found that the conductors who averaged daily over 500 steps up and down stairways on the buses had significantly less coronary artery disease than the drivers who were sedentary at their job all day. Furthermore, the drivers were much more likely to have a first coronary artery event that was fatal, while the conductors who had coronary artery problems were much more likely to have angina as their first sign rather than death. This is the first hard evidence of inactivity as a risk factor in atherosclerotic disease. Since then, this has been confirmed by many other studies.

Stress. A recent article from Harvard Medical School is thought-provoking. Nearly 4,000 people were interviewed within 30 days after suffering an acute myocardial infarction. Their anger, if any, during the 2 hours before the infarction was assessed on a standardized anger scale. They found that the risk of an acute myocardial infarction was more than 2-fold greater in people who recalled having had outbursts of anger, and that greater intensities of anger were associated with greater relative risks.

In their discussion they point out that outbursts of anger are associated with rises in blood pressure and outpouring of stress hormones.

Many years ago I had a disturbing but educational experience. I had been at a meeting in New York City and flew back to Indianapolis next to a middle-aged man I didn't know. We had a nice conversation and I got his name. It was a snowy blustery winter night and as I walked toward my car in the parking lot, I noticed a dark shadow on the snow. It was my traveling companion lying there and I immediately found that he was pulseless. CPR had recently been invented and I had learned how to do it, so I went to work while calling to some other passersby to call for help. Nothing that I or the rescue squad could do saved him. The next morning, I found his number in the phone book and called his wife to commiserate. She thanked me for trying to help him and told me that just a couple of days before he had gone to a cardiologist and gotten a clean bill of health. The message of this anecdote is the unpredictability of coronary occlusion. I am surmising that the plaque that was the culprit did not occlude enough to give the doctor a clue, until suddenly it ruptured, a clot formed and enough occlusion ensued to start ventricular fibrillation and death. And probably, the exertion of walking to the car in that cold wind contributed an element of coronary artery spasm. I assume you all are aware of the fact that shoveling snow on a cold day at our age is inviting trouble because the combination of effort and cold brings on coronary artery spasm.

At this point, it is useful to say a word about the importance of getting immediate help if you experience any of the warning symptoms. Besides the ones I have already enumerated, I should re-emphasize that if you already have been diagnosed as having angina and you get an attack of angina that lasts 10 minutes without the expected relief it is time to call for help.

Next we will consider modes of treatment of acute myocardial infarction. Here is what ideally will happen if you call for help and it comes quickly. The ambulance attendants will check and ensure that your heart is beating and you have a decent level of blood pressure. If not, they have an external defibrillator and know how to use it. If you need oxygen they can give it to you by mask or nasal tubes. At some point soon, either in the ambulance or at the ER, you will probably be given some aspirin to stop the clotting. And possibly an injection of a clot-dissolving drug. For pain and to dilate arterioles all over the body so the heart works less, you may get nitroglycerin under the tongue. If the pain is too severe, they can inject morphine under the skin. When you get to the ER, the ambulance has already called ahead and they will be ready for you. Time is of the essence, and the hope is to save as much of the compromised heart muscle as possible.

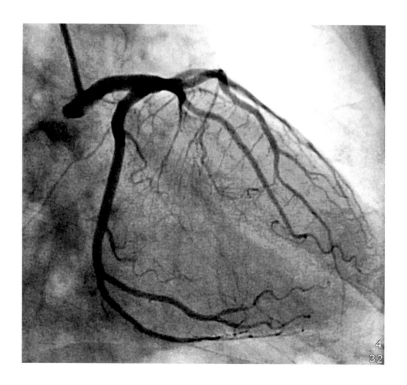

Fig. 8.2 A normal coronary arteriogram.

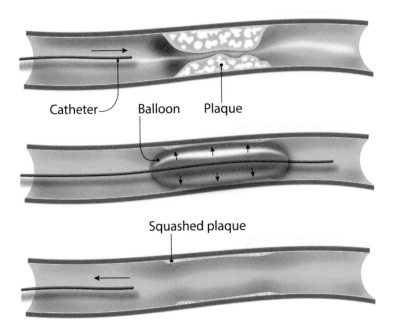

Fig. 8.3 Atherosclerotic plaque is stretched and dilated with a balloon.

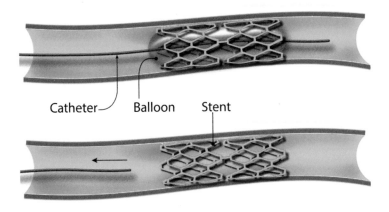

Fig. 8.4 A stent is inserted to maintain the dilation.

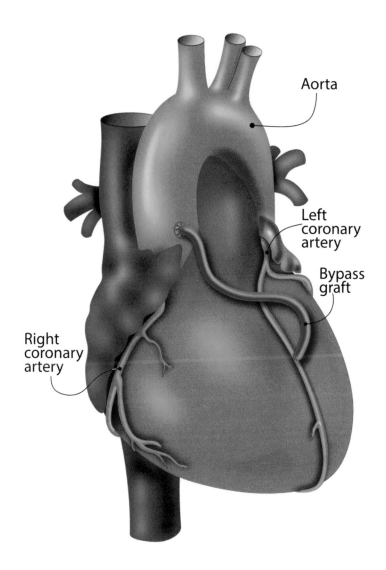

Fig. 8.5 A single coronary artery bypass graft.

As quickly as possible you will be taken to a catheterization lab where under local anesthesia a catheter will be inserted and passed through an artery to the root of the aorta and contrast will be injected into each coronary artery. This will map out whatever blockages there are (Fig. 8.2) and the next step is to balloon-dilate those areas (Fig. 8.3) and possibly insert stents (Fig. 8.4) to keep the dilated areas open. If needed some of the drugs we have talked about earlier for the treatment of congestive heart failure and/or high blood pressure will be started. An alternative which is harder to organize quickly is bypass surgery (Fig. 8.5) in which a length of vein is harvested and used as a graft between the aorta or one of its branches and the coronary artery beyond the blockage, or, if necessary, to bypass several blockages, in what is called triple or quadruple bypass. Before discharge from the hospital you will be instructed in lifestyle changes to prevent another attack and perhaps will be enrolled in a cardiac rehab program. This is a carefully programmed set of gradually increasing aerobic exercises.

Sometimes emergency treatment is required for an expanding or ruptured aneurysm, usually of the aorta. Again, the symptom that calls attention to the emergency is usually pain, and where the pain is depends on what branch arteries are compromised. Again, the treatment is either surgical, by opening the region in question or interventional by percutaneous, transarterial insertion of a plastic graft. (Fig. 8.6)

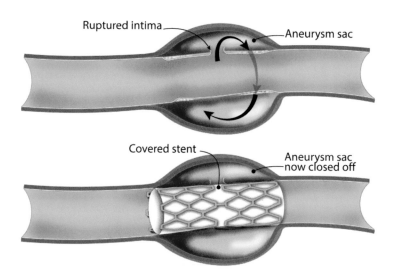

Fig. 8.6 Mechanism of development of an arterial aneurysm and method of treatment by insertion and expansion of a plastic graft which incorporates a stent.

9

LIFE STYLE CHANGES

In this chapter, my daughter Andrea takes over and will discuss fat, diet, obesity and lifestyle and how these all fit in the context of atherosclerosis.

I'm not a doc like my dad, but because of him, I've always been interested in cardio-respiratory fitness. When I retired from practice of law, I became a certified fitness professional. I teach fitness classes and have private clients. Because almost all my students and clients want to lose weight, I've become interested in the science and social policy of fat. We live in an obesogenic environment, with fast food joints and salty-fatty-sugary snack foods on almost every corner. At the same time, we unabashedly shame people who are overweight. Advising people simply to "eat less and move more" doesn't work for everyone over the long haul. Instead, I like to think that the more we know about the fat in our bodies and the fat in our food, the more effective our weight management efforts can be and the kinder we can be to ourselves and others.

In this chapter, we are going to look at why we need body fat; how the different kinds of fat cells function in our bodies; how body fat (and cholesterol) and the fat we eat affects our cardiovascular health. We'll sum up with some simple tips on how to manage weight and protect our cardiovascular health.

First and foremost, fat cells – adipocytes - have a major role in storing and releasing energy as we need it. Remember that Mother Nature did not anticipate that we would be living in a time when there was a Quickie Mart around every corner. Instead, she was preparing our bodies for a famine or for the day when we had to hide in a cave from a saber toothed tiger. Even now, Mother Nature wants to be sure that we have some slow releasing energy from stored fat in order to keep alive. Adipose (fat) tissue also cushions us when we fall and insulates us from cold. Fat cells help protect nerve tissue, and they send important messages relating to appetite and metabolism to other parts of the body. So, for example, when our fat stores are full, the fat cells send out a hormone called leptin (from the Greek for thin). Leptin tells the brain, and the brain tells us that we don't have to run out the door to continue our hunting and gathering – we're "full." The takeaway is that some body fat is necessary for healthy living.

Fat enters our bodies when we eat. The fats in our food are broken down into molecules in the intestines, absorbed into the gut wall and re-assembled into triglycerides – the fat that our bodies use for energy once our sugar stores are exhausted. Because the triglycerides can't travel through the bloodstream by themselves – oil and water don't mix – large lipoproteins called chylomicrons are released from the gut wall to carry the triglycerides, along with cholesterol and some other substances, into the bloodstream. Fat cells and muscle cells both can recognize the chylomicron package and send out an enzyme called lipase to pick up the fat. The chylomicrons eventually shrink and end up in the liver (see Figure 9.1).

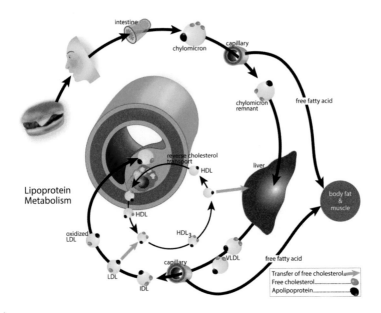

Fig. 9.1 Lipoprotein metabolism

Scientists so far have identified four different kinds of fat cells in our bodies, each with a somewhat different function.

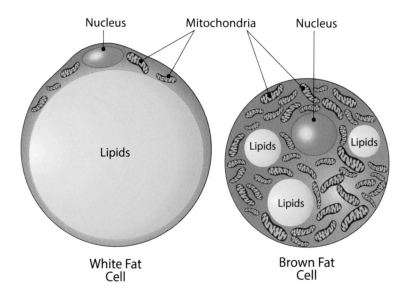

Fig. 9.2 White fat cells are structurally very different from brown. Since they are metabolically active, the brown fat cells have many more mitochondria. White fat cells have a single lipid compartment, brown have several.

First are the white subcutaneous fat cells that form the "pinch an inch" fat just under our skin. In addition to storing energy from food, subcutaneous fat acts as an energy absorber to cushion us – it's even been found in one study to protect against abdominal injuries in car crashes. Subcutaneous fat is benign. So, for example, removal of subcutaneous fat through liposuction does not appear to have any health benefits in terms of blood pressure, cholesterol levels or insulin sensitivity. And there actually is preliminary research suggesting that subcutaneous fat might be protective in some people against atherosclerosis.

Cellulite simply is normal subcutaneous fat that is constricted by connective tissue, which causes the skin to pucker. People may think it's unsightly, but it's not a health issue.

Second, we have the white fat cells that surround our hearts, intestines and other vital organs – visceral fat. Scientists just discovered recently that visceral fat actually differs in structure and genetic origin from subcutaneous fat. Visceral fat deposits also are protected by a membrane – a mesothelium – which is something previously not thought to exist in adipose tissue. The mesothelium surrounds and protects the visceral fat cell deposits in the abdomen – making them like neat little organs. Visceral fat also operates like an endocrine gland, sending hormonal messages out to other parts of the body to help regulate metabolism.

We need some visceral fat for good health, but too much visceral fat increases the risk of certain cancers (scientists are not yet sure why), non-alcoholic fatty liver disease, type 2 diabetes and Alzheimer's disease. Abdominal obesity also is associated strongly with high blood pressure, stroke, chronic low-grade inflammation and coronary artery disease.

Visceral fat is called a silent killer, because you might have a lot of visceral fat, but not look fat on the outside. Scale weight is not a good measure of visceral fat; nor is BMI (Body Mass Index). A simple way to assess visceral fat is waist measurement. A waist measurement over 33" for women carries some health risk; over 35" is considered high risk. For men, risk increases with waist size over 40".

The good news is that visceral fat disappears almost twice as fast as subcutaneous fat when we apply exercise and dietary changes.

Recently, scientists have been focusing on two other kinds of fat in our bodies – the brown and the beige. Until a few years ago, it was believed that only babies had brown and beige fat. Although brown and beige fat cells are genetically distinct from one another, they share the characteristic that they both are metabolically active. That is, brown and beige fat cells generate heat, thus using energy, i.e., calories, unlike our white fat cells that mostly store energy. It was thought that as we grow up, we didn't need brown or beige fat because we can shiver to keep warm. Recent studies however found that adults do have brown fat and beige fat, mostly in our necks, and that some people have more than others.

Because brown and beige fat use energy, there's a lot of research going on in how to convert white fat to brown fat or beige – a breakthrough that could be the magic bullet in the obesity wars. Scientists have identified a hormone called irisin that is created during muscle contractions. With muscle contraction – which could be exercise as well as shivering - irisin travels through the blood to white fat cells, where it actually transforms white fat cells into brown fat. This has caused some scientists to speculate that central heating has been one contributor to the current obesity crisis. Keep in mind that these metabolically active brown cells are our friends, and that exercise (not just shivering) may increase our store of them – a good reason, among the many good reasons, to exercise!

Those are the 4 types of fat cells – now, here's some general information about fat:

Contrary to the old saw, muscle does not weigh more than fat. Muscle just is denser and more compact than fat, so it takes up less room. So if you lose fat and gain muscle, you might not see much of a change in scale weight, but you will see a change in the size and shape of your body.

Another old saw is that you can change fat into muscle with diet and exercise. In fact, muscle cells are muscle cells and fat cells are fat cells: they have different functions and different genetic origins. It's not possible to convert one to another.

When one undertakes a weight-loss program, the goal should be not only to lose visceral fat, but also to maintain and actually add muscle. Muscle cells, like our friends the brown fat cells, are metabolically active. They use more calories, even when we are at rest, than white fat.

White fat cells can expand from three to six times their size. Once a fat cell has reached its maximum storage capacity, we have hyperplasia, i.e., it makes new fat cells. It's important to know that once a fat cell is made, it doesn't go away. It may shrink, but it never disappears. True, one can remove fat cells with liposuction or kill them off with "Cool Sculpting." However, without serious lifestyle changes in terms of diet and exercise, our bodies simply will create new fat cells to replace the ones that were removed.

White fat cells are replaced at the rate of about 10% per year in adults. So about every 10 years, we replace our old fat cells with new ones – but the numbers remain steady. Even if one loses weight, those fat cells still are there, crying out hormonally to be filled up again with stored fat. The takeaway here is that it's better to never gain weight than it is to gain weight and then try to lose it. Realize, also, that Mother Nature fears for our safety when we lose fat, because she can't distinguish between famine and extreme dieting. If our body goes into famine mode, she will defend mightily against fat loss. The result can be "yo-yo" dieting, where one sticks to a rigid eating plan for a while, then falls off the wagon, gaining back the weight lost and often more. People who have had long-term weight-loss success recognize this, and develop sensible eating plans and exercise routines that they can live with over the long haul.

Finally, despite the ads on late night TV for magic ab belts or the "flat belly diet" plans touted in magazines, one cannot spot reduce, either by eating certain special foods or by doing a ton of abdominal exercises. Again, successful weight maintenance requires finding an eating plan and exercise routine that one can live with over the long haul.

Now we turn to a brief look at cholesterol. This waxy, fat-like substance is necessary for normal cell function and repair. It helps us make vitamin D; helps make the bile salts that we need for digestion; and performs many other essential functions in our bodies.

Cholesterol is made in our livers. We also eat cholesterol from animal products, most notably meat and dairy. The liver generally does a pretty good job of regulating our cholesterol levels, so if we eat more cholesterol, the liver will adjust and make less. Problems arise when we take in too much dietary fat and cholesterol or if, for other reasons – genetics, certain diseases - the body makes more cholesterol than the cells can process.

Cholesterol isn't water-soluble, so it can't go through the bloodstream on its own. It travels, like the triglycerides, in chylomicrons and other lipoprotein packets (see Fig. 9.3).

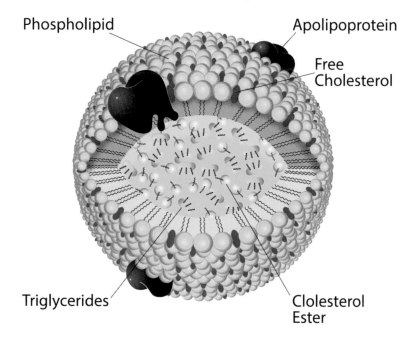

Chylomicron

Fig. 9.3 A chylomicron

Low-density lipoprotein – LDL (the so-called "bad

cholesterol") – is not bad in and of itself. LDL is the lipoprotein that carries cholesterol from the liver out to the body, where it's needed for cell repair and other functions.

Each LDL particle has one apolipoprotein B, and it's the APO B that actually gets stuck to the artery wall. Family practice Doctor Spencer Nadolsky (http://drspencer.com) explains it as cholesterol is the cargo and apoB is the tugboat, and they travel though your arteries like a barge on a river. The trouble starts when the apoB tug crashes into the sides of the river – the inner walls of your arteries. It sticks, and it starts the inflammatory process that results in the formation of the plaques that contribute to artery disease.

LDL particles vary in size and density. The smaller, denser particles are the most dangerous because they are better able to get into the artery walls. The smaller particles also seem to be associated with other risk factors: low high-density lipoprotein numbers (HDL - the so-called "good cholesterol"), high triglycerides, high blood sugar – and not surprisingly– visceral fat.

Some people actually have a discordance between LDL cholesterol levels and the LDL particle numbers. So you could have low LDL measurement, but lots of the small dense particles, thus falsely believe your heart disease risk is low; or you could have high LDL and big fluffy LDL particles, and falsely believe your risk of heart disease is higher than it is. Now there is advanced lipid testing that actually measures the amount of apo B (which gives you information on your particle size and number) and this test comes in handy in these cases of discordance. When it can be made cost-effective, this test may become the standard.

HDL carries cholesterol from the cells through the bloodstream back to the liver for reuse. Each HDL particle is carried on an apolipoprotein A particle. Apo A's are believed to actually protect against atherosclorosis.

Triglyceride numbers simply reflect the amount of fat stored in the body. High triglycerides are linked to heart disease, especially where there's low HDL.

In cases of dyslipidemia – abnormal amounts of cholesterol or fat in the blood – lifestyle changes, such as eating healthy and exercising generally are the first line of defense. Statins, a class of drugs that are given to patients with bad cholesterol numbers, work by inhibiting an enzyme that controls cholesterol production in the liver. Statins were in the news in November of 2013, when the

American Heart Association and the American College of Cardiology published new guidelines for lowering cholesterol, along with an online calculator (downloadable at http://my.americanheart.org) meant to help doctors assess patients' risks. There is much controversy about this calculator, because some medical professionals believe that it overestimates risk. More will be revealed in time, but the bottom line is that each physician needs to look at each individual to determine whether some kind of intervention is needed. This may be either lifestyle changes alone or lifestyle changes in combination with statins or other medications.

It also is worth noting that we need much more information on how statins affect women, because most of the research on these drugs has been done with male subjects. Also, a 12-year study completed in 2014 showed that people who use statins gradually increase their consumption of fat and calories. We now need to look at whether statins increase appetite or whether they give people taking them a false sense of security. But most experts would agree that taking statins cannot replace the benefits of a healthy lifestyle. The two must go hand in hand.

So to sum up this section: We need some body fat

and we need some cholesterol. However, too much body fat, particularly visceral fat, can have serious health consequences, even if it's in a skinny body. Some argue that it is possible to be fat and fit. But there's a recent study that looked at 14,000 metabolically healthy adults with no known cardiovascular disease. Looking at their coronary artery calcium scores, the obese individuals in the study were more likely to have early stage plaque build-up than their normal weight counterparts. The recommendation from the study was that all overweight individuals should be counseled to improve their diet and exercise habits, even if they have no symptoms of cardiovascular disease.

The good news is that, even for an overweight person, a mere five percent weight loss can produce medically measurable beneficial results, so any amount of weight loss is helpful if one is overweight or obese.

We turn now to the fat we eat and how it affects our health.

There are three macronutrients: fat, carbohydrates and protein. We need a balance of all of them to live.

Like the fat in our bodies, the fat we eat is not *per se* our enemy. We need dietary fat to absorb fat-soluble vitamins like A and E, to help maintain healthy skin and hair and for brain health. Dietary fats also increase the time needed to empty food from our stomachs, so they provide a sense of fullness, which can help limit the amount of food we eat.

Fats have a very high energy yield – a gram of fat has nine calories versus four calories per gram of carbohydrate or protein. So for example, a serving of almonds – just 24 nuts – is 165 calories.[1] Now, almonds are densely nutritious; they contain good fats, some carbohydrates for quick energy and some protein to help build and repair muscle. That handful of almonds is a beautiful package of food, but it's possible to quickly nibble up too much of a good thing! Just be aware that one's total daily fat intake should be somewhat less than 30 percent of one's total daily caloric intake. It helps to be particularly mindful of the amounts of fat in the form of butter, salad dressing (a tablespoon of olive oil has about 120 calories), grated cheese and the like that one is adding to food. Moderation is key.

Some fats are healthier than others, and some are

---

[1] For someone who needs only 1600-2000 calories a day to maintain his/her weight, several big handfuls of nuts can add up to the equivalent of a meal.

hazardous to our heart health.

Saturated fats are the dietary fats that come mainly from animal sources such as meat and dairy products. For a long time, saturated fats were considered the major villain in coronary artery disease. That started a no-fat and lo-fat trend in food production and marketing that some scientists and food experts now think is partly responsible for our current obesity epidemic. At the height of the no-fat craze, people often replaced satisfying, nutritious real foods with refined carbohydrates – pasta, rice and bread and sugary snacks - because they were marketed as being lo-fat or having no cholesterol and thus "healthy." A lot of the new information is that in fact eating some saturated fats may be good for us.

The so-far undisputed good guys of the dietary fat world are the monounsaturated fats that are found in various oils: olive, peanut, grapeseed oil, safflower, sesame, walnut, flaxseed, sunflower and some others. They also are found in avocados and almonds, peanut butter, dark chocolate, whole olives and to some extent in red meat and whole milk products. Olive oil in particular gets a lot of praise for its heart health effects – there's a chemical in freshly pressed, extra virgin olive oil that acts as a natural anti-inflammatory, it's akin to what's in aspirin. Again, while these fats are healthy to eat, they are densely caloric and should be consumed in moderation.

The polyunsaturated fats found in fish, whole grain wheat, bananas, walnuts, hemp seed and some vegetable oils also are good guys. However, there's some question about the healthiness of the highly refined polyunsaturates - soy oil, corn oil and cottonseed oils - that are common in fast food and processed foods. It's been found that as much as 20 percent of the calories in the typical American diet come from soybean oil. The processed polyunsaturates are problematic because they are high in omega-6 fatty acids, unlike unprocessed whole foods such as walnuts, flax, sardines and anchovies and avocados, that have lots of omega-3 fatty acids. We need both omega 3s and omega 6s, but they need to be in a certain balance. Our typical American diet tends to be very high in omega 6s, another possible cause for the obesity epidemic.

The evil-doers of the fat world are the trans fats. When unsaturated vegetable oils are treated with hydrogen – hydrogenated – they usually turn into trans fats. Fully or partially hydrogenated vegetable oils commonly are used in processed foods – because they retard spoilage -- and used in movie popcorn and restaurant frying, although a lot of jurisdictions have outlawed selling food fried in trans fats. Trans fats are the primary fats that are implicated in cardiovascular disease. Trans fats alone may account for at least 30,000 premature heart disease deaths in the US every year. When we eat products with trans fats, they drive up LDL and lower HDL more quickly than the other fats. They promote inflammation and insulin resistance. They've also recently been linked to incidence of depression – so those fast food meals aren't so happy after all.

In June, 2015, the US Food and Drug Administration (FDA) declared partially hydrogenated oils ("PHOs") not to be "generally recognized as safe", and gave food manufacturers three years to remove them from their products.

Note that a lot of prepared foods say they have no trans fats on the label, but food manufacturers don't have to admit that there are trans fats in the product if there are less than a prescribed amount per serving. That means that if you eat more than a "serving" according to the food label, you may be ingesting some trans fat. Plus, because trans fats have gotten such a bad reputation, food manufacturers have come up with an artificial alternative that may be just as bad: interesterified fats. Or they are substituting processed palm oil, which is a saturated fat that is not so healthy when it's gone through processing.

The bottom line is that we need fats in our diets, but our fats should come from whole foods – nuts, seeds, avocados, sardines and anchovies – because these give us not only the healthy fats, but all of the other nutrients – the antioxidants, proteins, fibers – that come in the whole food package. It is wise to steer away as much as possible from the hydrogenated and partially hydrogenated oils that are in many packaged foods and fast foods.

It's important to note here that, just because a product is labeled as "lo-fat" or "no-fat" does not mean that it's healthy. Fat, sugar and salt are what make foods tasty. Thus, if something doesn't have much fat, it probably has lots of salt or sweetener. Compare, for example, a peanut butter that is made just from peanuts, with no added salt or sugar, to one of its typical "reduced fat peanut spread" counterparts. The peanut spread boasts that it has 20% less fat than peanut butter, but still has that "fresh roasted peanut taste." Looking more closely at the nutritional label, however, the spread has only ten less calories per serving than the real peanut butter, but twice the sugars. There's a teaspoon of added sweetener to every tablespoon of peanut spread. Unlike the natural sugar from the peanuts, the reduced fat version is loaded with added simple sugars from corn syrup solids, table sugar and molasses. Although the front label claims that the spread has no trans fats, this is belied by the ingredients list that shows that the product contains fully hydrogenated vegetable oils from rapeseed and soy. The label also touts that the spread has no preservatives. Because of the trans fats, preservatives aren't needed. The real peanut butter has healthier unsaturated fat from the peanuts. Neither product has dietary cholesterol, because peanuts don't have cholesterol – they're from a plant. The takeaway is that one needs to be a savvy label reader – look at the nutrition label on the back, not the marketing slogans on the front.

As noted above, fats are one of three "macronutrients." We need all three, despite what some of the popular diet gurus may say. The other macronutrients are protein and carbohydrates. We need protein, chiefly to build and repair muscles. We need carbohydrates for quick energy and brain fuel. As with the fats, we can make healthy choices. For protein, look for the lean meats and fish and take some protein from plant sources such as legumes, nuts, seeds and whole grain. For carbohydrates, choose vegetables and fruit and whole grains. Avoid the simple sugars and refined carbohydrates that spike our blood sugar levels, then cause them to fall rapidly, so we crave that second doughnut.

Studies have shown that no popular "diet" has been proven to be better than another for long-term weight-loss maintenance, so pay no attention to all the diet fads and fancies. The only "food way" that's been proven to be heart healthy is the Mediterranean diet rich in fish, vegetables, fruits, nuts and olive oil. For another all-around heart healthy way to eat, check out the Harvard School of Public Health Healthy Eating Plate. (http://www.hsph.harvard.edu/nutritionsource/healthy-eating-plate).

Dietary fiber – found in vegetables, fruits and unrefined grains – also has been shown to reduce the risk of cardiovascular disease. A 2014 study suggested that the recommended fiber intake – 14 grams a day per each 1,000 calories consumed – helped prevent cardiovascular death in people who already had had a heart attack. There's a theory – that not all experts subscribe to – that fiber binds with cholesterol in the intestines and prevents it from being absorbed into the bloodstream. A lot of doctors think that a high fiber diet is heart-healthy simply because it substitutes plant-based foods for more fatty, high-calorie foods, i.e., if one eats oatmeal for breakfast, one isn't downing a platter of bacon, eggs and home fries.

If one wants to increase the fiber in one's diet, eat the whole vegetable or fruit. A Florida orange has 65 calories; 13 grams of sugar; and is 14% fiber. Compare this to a cup of orange juice, with its 112 calories; 20.8 grams of sugar; and only two percent is fiber. The fiber in the whole orange helps keep one's blood sugar steady and leaves one more satiated than the juice.

Note that a healthy diet may not result in weight loss. Any excess of food, no matter how healthy, will be stored, mostly as visceral fat.

This brings us to physical activity, heart health and fat loss.

The heart is a muscle and it needs to get exercise to stay healthy. The benefits of traditional cardiovascular exercise are legion – we all know it's good for us, so I won't belabor it. I hope that you can find some form of cardiovascular exercise that turns you on – whether it's walking, bike riding, swimming or dancing. You don't have to grind out 40 minutes or an hour on a treadmill. You can get a benefit from a minimum of ten minutes of cardiovascular exercise. Ten minutes of disco dancing in your kitchen while you're waiting for dinner to be ready can be a great cardio workout.

What we all need to focus more on is physical activity outside of exercise. In the previous chapter, Dad wrote about the London Transport study of the bus drivers and the conductors. The drivers sat all day, but the conductors were going up and down stairs of the double-deckers all day. The conductors had many fewer cardiac events, and the ones they had did not tend to be fatal.

What recent studies are finding is that sitting all day doubles the risk of heart disease, diabetes and obesity. Remember lipase - the enzyme that helps remove triglyceride-rich lipoproteins from the blood stream by transferring them to the muscles for energy or to HDL for disposal? When we sit, the action of lipase stops, so fat kind of just sits there in your bloodstream. People who sit a lot can see reductions in HDL of up to 22%.

In one study, researchers took plasma samples from the same person after eating the same meal. When the subject ate sitting down, the sample was cloudy with fat. When they ate standing up, the sample was clear. I'm not recommending eating standing up, but I do strongly recommend taking a walk after dinner instead of immediately hitting the couch to watch TV. What we need for heart health, in some ways more than traditional exercise, is to increase our non-exercise activity thermogenesis or NEAT. That's the physical activity we do outside of eating, sleeping and traditional "exercise." It includes walking, fidgeting, gardening, cooking, putting the dishes away after the meal – all the everyday activities that require energy expenditure above our basal metabolic rate (the energy we use at rest). Some easy ways to increase your daily NEAT are to walk around while using the phone; if you're waiting in line at the ATM, shift from one foot to the other; take the stairs instead of the elevator. If you're watching TV, get up and walk around (just not to the kitchen for a snack!) during the breaks. Those kinds of added movements don't take much effort, and you reap great rewards in terms of heart health and weight loss/maintenance. So remember to be a NEATnik and keep that lipase circulating.

In sum, neither our body fat nor the fats we eat are our enemies. We just need to leverage them to give us the most benefit. Exercise to harness the metabolic activity of our brown and beige fat cells. Get our dietary fats from moderate portions of whole foods, such as almonds, fish and real peanut butter, and limit our consumption of the processed fats that come in fast food meals and packaged pastries. Keep our lipase circulating, increase our

HDL cholesterol and use more calories by sneaking in non-exercise movement at every opportunity. Above all, kick the yo-yo dieting and find the heart-healthy eating and exercise routine that we can live with over the long haul.

10

HEART SURGERY AND INTERVENTIONAL CARDIOLOGY

This chapter is a historical account of the development of heart surgery and interventional cardiology.

The story starts in England in the 1890's when controversy first began in *The Lancet*, principal medical journal at the time as to whether or not it was ethical to tamper with the beating heart. Nevertheless, there were a few brave souls who felt obliged by emergency situations to proceed in spite of prevailing opinion.

In 1895, Dr. Axel Cappelen, in Kristiania (now Oslo), Norway, operated on a man who had been in a knife fight and was bleeding from multiple chest wounds, one of which had reached the heart. He entered the chest, ligated a bleeding coronary artery and the patient survived, only to die 2 days later of a myocardial infarction and infection. The following year Dr. Rehn of Frankfurt, Germany repaired a laceration of the right ventricle and the patient recovered. The next recorded event was that in 1912 Dr. Tuffier in Paris dilated a tight aortic valve while the heart was beating and the patient survived. In 1925, Dr. Souttar in France dilated a mitral valve in a beating heart. His colleagues pleaded with him to stop doing this and he complied. It must be understood that these plucky pioneers were operating at a time when opening the chest meant instant collapse of the lungs, which are held open normally by a slight vacuum in the pleural space around them.

By the early 1930s a couple of very simple but basic elements came together to make it possible to safely open the chest. These were the direct laryngoscope permitting easy insertion of a cuffed endotracheal tube, so that the anesthesiologist could administer gases that he or she chose under positive pressure, thus keeping the lungs inflated throughout the procedure.

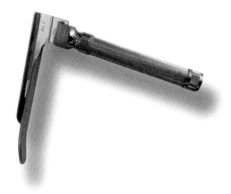

Fig. 10.1 Direct laryngoscope

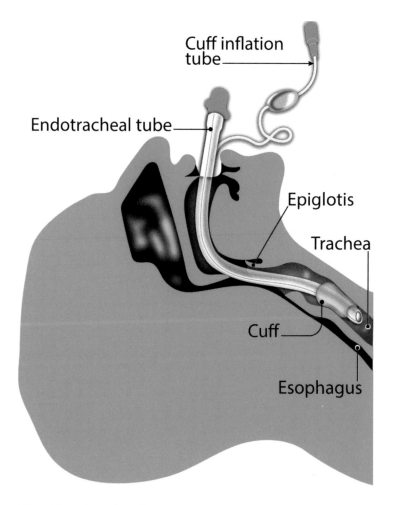

Cuff inflation tube

Endotracheal tube

Epiglotis

Trachea

Cuff

Esophagus

Fig. 10.2 A patient in whom an endotracheal tube has been passed into the trachea with the aid of a direct larygoscope after which the cuff on the tube has been inflated through the small tube, enabling the anesthetist to keep the lungs inflated with positive pressure.

World War II was a period of rapid advance in chest surgery, and cardiac surgery followed it closely. The first cardiac surgeries after the war were again, dilating obstructing valves in the beating heart with a gloved finger, sometimes with a tiny blade attached.

The next developments were in the area of congenital heart disease. The ductus arteriosus is a necessary structure in the fetus. It is a channel between the descending aorta and the pulmonary artery that permits blood to bypass the uninflated lungs. It has special contractile muscle in its walls that causes it to close in the higher oxygen environment of the newborn. If it does not close, blood constantly recirculates in the lungs in amounts determined mainly by how large is the remaining opening.

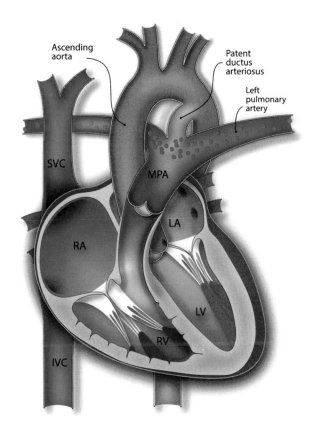

Fig. 10.3 a fairly large patent ductus arteriosus

It was now possible, at low risk, to close the ductus surgically, first by a simple ligature, a little later by transecting it and suturing the two ends using vascular surgical techniques that had been learned in the treatment of trauma in World War II.

The next congenital structure to be fixed surgically was coarctation of the aorta.

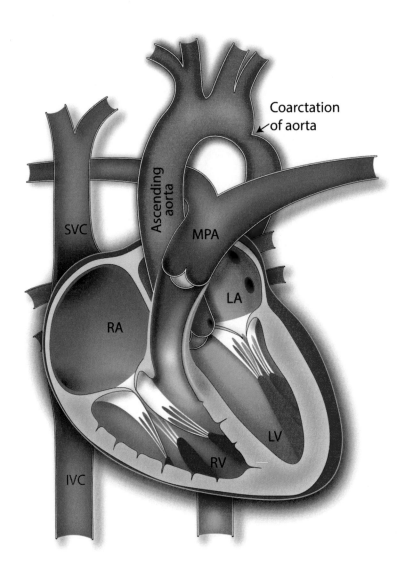

Fig. 10.4 Coarctation of the aorta

This constriction of the main artery is certainly counterproductive and can cause real problems, including congestive heart failure and hypertension in the arteries to the head and arms. It is thought to result when some of that contractile ductus tissue got misplaced a little in fetal life and caused the aorta to be narrowed. In this operation the surgeon removes the constriction, then sews the cut ends back together, which even better demonstrates the ability to cut and sew arteries together that had been developed in the war.

That skill was put to good use in 1944 in an operation which really was magical and put the fields of pediatric cardiology and cardiac surgery on the map. At that time there were thousands of babies and children, even a few adults, who were blue rather than pink because of a group of malformations shown here.

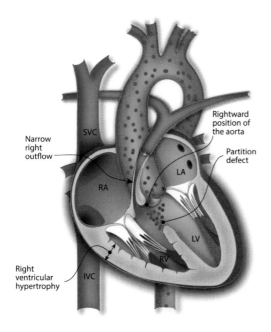

Fig. 10.5 Tetralogy of Fallot

It is called Tetralogy of Fallot because of four abnormalities close together in the developing heart. These are a narrowing of the outflow of the right ventricle, a defect high on the partition between the two ventricles, a rightward position of the aorta and hypertrophy of the right ventricle so that it is of a thickness more like that of the left ventricle. Unoxygenated blood that can't pass into the lungs because of the narrowing of the pulmonary outflow passes across the defect into the aorta and is recirculated to the body. The patients were a pathetic bunch who had no exercise tolerance at all, were often dyspneic at rest and spent much of their waking lives in a squatting position. Their fingers and toes were clubbed.

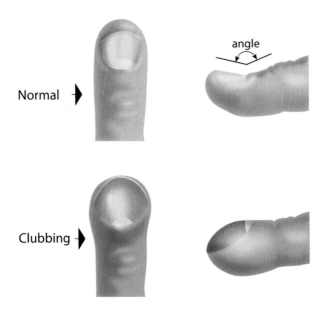

Fig. 10.6 Clubbing

There was a pediatrician named Helen Taussig on the full time staff at Johns Hopkins who had been assigned to head a newly established Cardiac Clinic. In those days, the 1940s, her main job was taking care of patients with rheumatic fever and the heart disease that results from it, mainly a scarring, which affects the heart valves. But she also accumulated considerable experience observing blue babies. She observed that after birth, as long as the characteristic murmur of patent ductus persisted, these babies remained pink; but as soon as the ductus closed, they got blue. She reasoned that the protective effect of the patent ductus was increased blood flow to the lungs, bypassing the narrowing of the pulmonary artery that restricted the flow. Perhaps a surgical connection from the aorta to the pulmonary artery, essentially an artificial ductus, would help these patients.

She took her idea to Alfred Blalock, Head of Surgery at Hopkins. He was not enthusiastic as he had recently taken the job, having come from Vanderbilt University Medical School. At Vanderbilt he had had the good fortune of hiring as a cleaning boy in his surgical lab a black woodworker who was a would-be surgeon. This highly endowed and inventive fellow named Vivien Thomas became his valued lab technician.

Blalock brought Vivien with him from Vanderbilt. He assigned to Vivien the task of making an animal preparation that mimicked tetralogy and then attempting to cure it with the operation suggested by Dr. Taussig. It was quite a job, but Vivien understood its importance even more than Blalock did and after months in the lab, he proved the validity of the idea, actually detaching a subclavian artery from the dog's front paw and implanting it in the pulmonary artery. Taussig followed events in the animal lab and soon began to urge Blalock to try it. He finally agreed to perform the first blue baby operation in 1944. He refused to operate until he had Vivien at his side in the OR. Taussig of course was also in the room for that first operation. Dr. Ruth Whittemore was a fellow intern in Pediatrics with me at Yale in 1942-43. When I went into the service in World War II Ruth went to Hopkins and finished her pediatric residency. She was an assistant resident in pediatrics when that first blue baby was operated on and stayed up all night with the child. The operation was a great success and Ruth was so thrilled with the whole thing that she stayed on at Hopkins as Taussig's first fellow. Five years later, when I had returned from the war and finished my pediatric residency at Yale, I was asked to be Ruth's first fellow, as she returned to New Haven to start a specialized Pediatric Cardiac Clinic like

Taussig's. We started the first cardiac catheterization lab devoted to children there at Yale and soon, with the help of surgeons trained under Blalock, were taking care of many blue babies. Availability of surgical amelioration opened the floodgates and these kids started coming from everywhere. The specialty that I would spend the rest of my career on had been born.

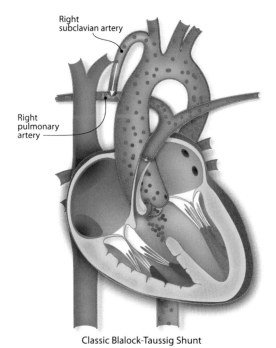

Classic Blalock-Taussig Shunt

Fig. 10.7 The operation completed. Right subclavian artery has been connected to right pulmonary artery.

The right subclavian artery has been severed and reconnected to the right pulmonary artery, thus adding to the amount of mixed venous blood traversing the lungs and increasing systemic arterial oxygen.

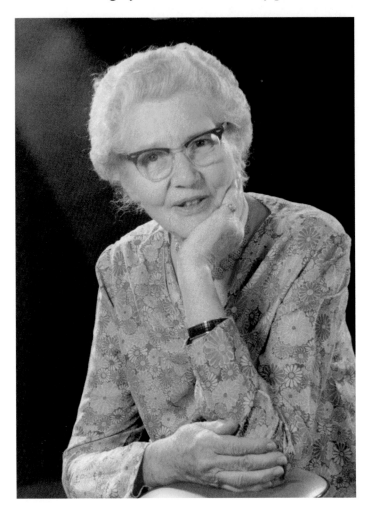

Fig. 10.8 Helen B. Taussig, M.D., the pediatrician who envisioned the concept and became the founder of pediatric cardiology.

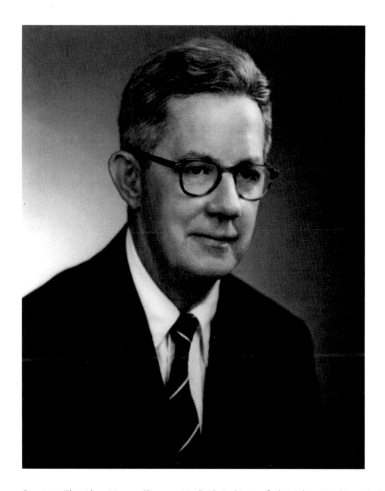

Fig. 10.9 Alfred Blalock M.D., the surgeon.

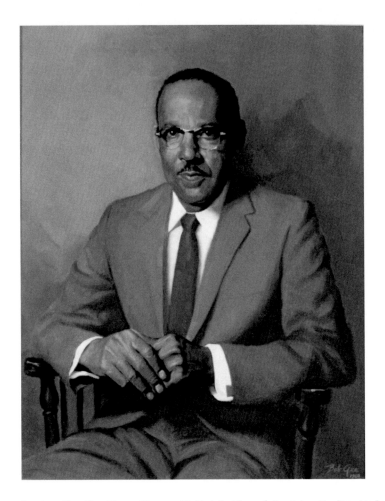

Courtesy The Alan Mason Chesney Medical Archives of the Johns Hopkins Medical Institutions.

Fig. 10.10 Vivien Thomas, the technician who enabled it all.

I went on from there to head Pediatric Cardiology at Indiana University and then at University of Southern California. Over the next three decades I was in a position to watch the further developments in cardiac surgery at first hand. While I am not a surgeon myself, it is the job of the pediatric cardiologist to accurately diagnose the patient's problem and present the surgeon with a road map and suggestions as to the best remedy. The Blalock-Taussig shunt procedure was outside the heart but soon surgeons were experimenting with procedures that eventually led to open heart surgery on a quiet heart. The heart-lung bypass machine did not appear overnight. First came some attempts to operate quickly on a heart stopped during deep hypothermia. This was soon abandoned because of the risk of brain damage. Next came a few procedures in Minneapolis in 1954 when a parent was hooked up with his or her child for a short period so that the child's heart could be excluded from the circulation, opened and fixed. This also was soon abandoned because of dangerous complications for the parent but it certainly stimulated others to push ahead. John Kirklin of the Mayo Clinic had built a replica of the membrane oxygenator developed by Dr. Gibbon of Philadelphia. At the same time Dr. DeWall of the University of Minnesota team invented a simple bubble oxygenator. In 1955, two hospitals a few miles apart in Minnesota, were doing the only open heart surgery in the world. The rest of the world's cardiac surgeons followed as quickly as they could and in less than a year, the so called heart-lung machine was in wide use.

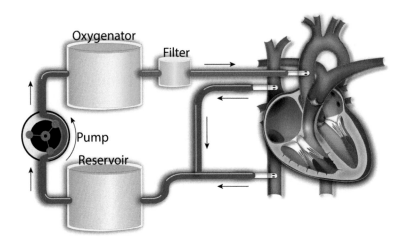

Fig. 10.11 The "Heart-lung machine".

Its basic elements are a pump and an oxygenator. Blood is sucked in through the two tubes in the vena cava above and below the heart. It is pumped through the oxygenator and returned to the aorta above the heart.

Heart-lung bypass permitted lengthy procedures like the complicated repair of a common arterial trunk shown in the next three pages.

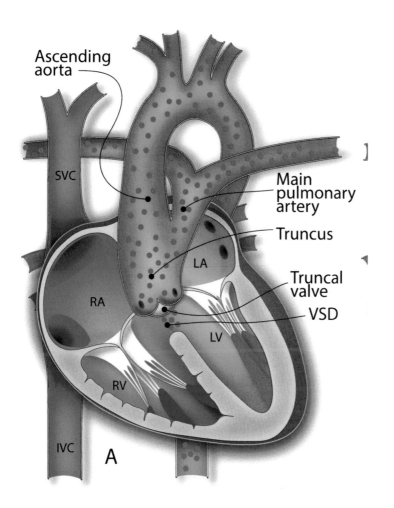

Ascending aorta

SVC

Main pulmonary artery

Truncus

Truncal valve

VSD

LA

RA

LV

RV

IVC

A

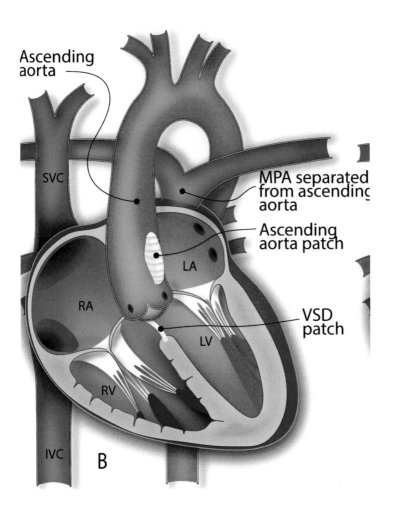

Ascending aorta

SVC

MPA separated from ascending aorta

Ascending aorta patch

LA

RA

VSD patch

LV

RV

IVC

B

164

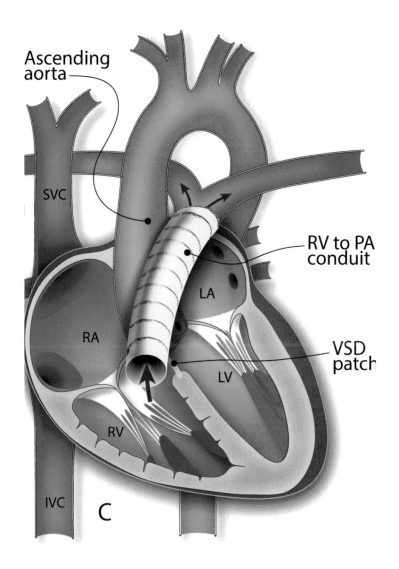

Fig. 10.12 Common arterial trunk (A) and its stepwise repair (B and C)

A. The pulmonary artery arises as a branch of the aorta, the two having never divided in fetal development. A large ventricular septal defect underlies the common trunk B. The pulmonary artery is detached and the defect in the trunk is closed with a patch. C. The repair is completed by connecting the right ventricle to the pulmonary artery and closing the ventricular septal defect.

A few years later, the bypass procedure for coronary artery blockage came along, benefiting huge numbers of adults (Fig. 8.5, page 117). It was at first usually done with cardiopulmonary bypass and a quiet heart, though more recently with the heart continuing to pump and just immobilizing enough of it to make the necessary connections. Robot-assisted surgery on the heart is being increasingly utilized, as well.

In 1966 my fellow pediatric cardiologist and good friend, Bill Rashkind of Philadelphia Childrens Hospital, came out with a solution for one of the most troubling and difficult of all congenital heart disease, complete transposition of the aorta and pulmonary artery.

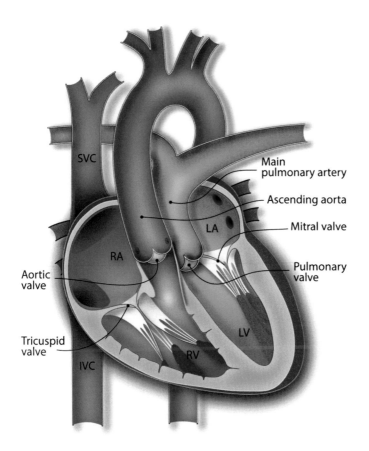

Fig. 10.13 Complete transposition of the great arteries.

Unoxygenated blood from the right ventricle is returned to the body. Oxygenated blood is pumped back into the lungs.

As you can see, if the normal changes occurred at birth, namely, closure of the ductus and closure of the opening between the atria, the infant with transposition was doomed. What Bill did, using both imagination and sheer guts, was to pass a catheter with a balloon on it across the atrial septum, inflate the balloon and yank it back vigorously so as to tear the tissue covering the atrial septum and thereby greatly increase the interchange between the pulmonary and systemic circuits. The baby's systemic arterial oxygen level increased significantly instantly!

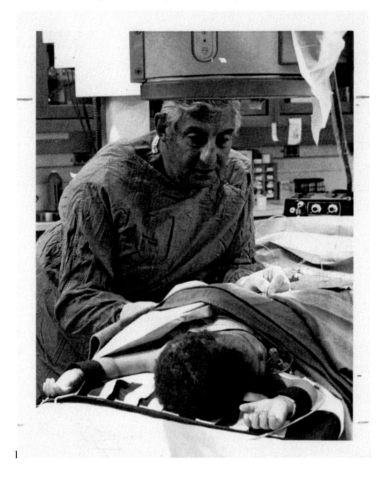

Fig. 10.14 William J. Rashkind MD performing a cardiac catheterization

Later, surgical technique advanced to the point where surgeons were fully repairing transposition in infancy by transplanting the aorta and pulmonary artery to their normal positions.. However, in places where such surgical ability is unavailable, the balloon atrial septostomy continues to save babies' lives. Even more important is the fact that this was the first procedure in a subsequent series of developments in the new field of interventional cardiology, which we will now discuss.

Once again, Bill Rashkind was on the front of a wave. Sometime in 1981, he phoned me and asked if I or one of my associates would like to come to Philadelphia to spend a few hours in his animal lab, trying to close atrial septal defects with a catheter-borne gadget he had been developing in collaboration with the Franklin Institute. I agreed and two of us went from Los Angeles to Philadelphia. He had prepared some calves with artificially created atrial septal defects and about 6 of us friends of his from childrens' hospitals around the country were given the privilege of closing the defects with his instrument. It worked! What a thrill!

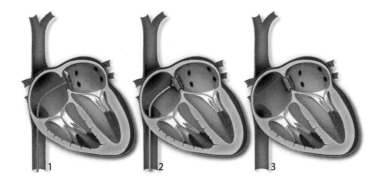

Fig. 10.15 Shows how a catheter-borne 2-part device can close an atrial septal defect.

Here are a few other uses of interventional cardiology.

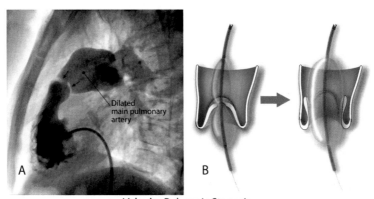

Valvular Pulmonic Stenosis
A, Lateral view, the arrows show the doming pulmonary valve. B, schematic of pulmonary balloon valvuloplasty

Fig. 10.16 Dilating stuck valves. This is an angiocardiogram showing a stenotic pulmonic valve. It is thickened and domed in systole with a jet pointing into the post-stenotically dilated pulmonary artery. The strong balloon, inflated to high pressure, breaks open the valve.

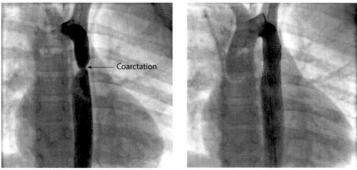

Coarctation of Aorta
A, before dilatation. B, after stent placement

Fig. 10.17 Dilating coarctation of the aorta

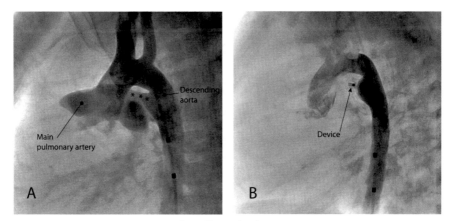

Patent Ductus Arteriosus
A, before occlusion, the asterisks show the patent ductus. B, after device occlusion

Fig. 10.18, Closing patent ductus arteriosus with a catheter-borne device.

Nowadays, as we saw in Chapter 8, occluded coronary arteries are being dilated and stented, and massive arterial aneurymal dilations and dissections are being fixed with tubes that can be compressed and deployed through catheters into positions where they are needed. The latest development in this progression is the complete deployable artificial valve. So far, these are most successful in the pulmonic position, where the stress is least, but percutaneous solutions are becoming available for mitral regurgitation and also for aortic stenosis (Fig. 10.19), a growing problem as the population ages.

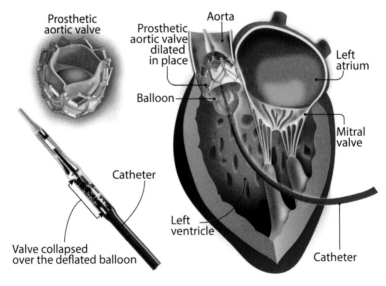

Fig. 10.19 A device for replacing an aortic valve made to fit within a catheter and deployed to show both valve and surrounding stent. In this case the valve is passed through the chest wall. A needle is inserted through skin and muscle into the apex of the enlarged heart and into the left ventricular cavity. A guide wire with a soft tip is passed through the needle and up into the aorta through the stenotic valve.

The catheter carrying the prosthetic valve is passed over the guide wire to the site of the valve where it is released while being expanded to remain in position. The alternative is to insert the needle, guide wire and catheter through the skin into the femoral artery at the groin and pass the catheter up the aorta, around the arch to the valve site and release the prosthetic valve there under pressure.

This concludes our journey. We have covered a lot of territory, and I hope for the reader it has been a fascinating adventure.

GLOSSARY

Aerobic exercise: Exercise at low enough intensity that demands for oxygen are satisfied and lactic acid is not built up. In contrast is anaerobic exercise which can be either at a higher intensity such as a 400 M race which is both aerobic and anaerobic or a 100 M dash in which the runner does not breathe appreciably for the few seconds of the event.

Angina pectoris: "squeezing of the chest" usually chest pain spreading to shoulders or arms, along with nausea, pallor, and cold sweats.

Angiocardiography: a series of x-ray pictures of the heart or vessels taken during injection of radiopaque contrast medium into the blood stream.

Arrhythmia (or dysrhythmia): any form of cardiac rhythm abnormality.

Atherosclerosis; synonyms: arteriosclerosis, hardening of the arteries: a disease of the arteries due to buildup of plaques formed of cholesterol and other substances that can lead to narrowing or complete occlusion.

Atria: right and left upper storage chambers.

Atypical angina: vague pain in back or neck, perhaps with nausea.

Bradycardia: excessively slow heart rate.

Cardiac output: volume per minute pumped by the heart.

Cardiomyopathy: disease of heart muscle, usually either dilated (too thin) or hypertrophic (too thick).

Diastole: the phase of the cardiac cycle when the heart muscle relaxes.

Dyspnea: breahlessness.

Electrode: a wire or similar conductor that picks up or transmits an electrical signal.

Fibrillation: When heart chambers contract constantly without filling or emptying, contributing no strength to contraction.

Heart attack: An inexact lay term that includes many possible causes of sudden onset of cardiac difficulty. The most common example is the sudden occlusion of a coronary artery.

Heart failure: Short for Congestive heart failure, in which the heart chronically falls short of carrying its load, so that excess fluid builds up in either the pulmonary circuit or the systemic circuit or both.

Infarction: death of tissue due to loss of blood supply.

Ischemia: loss of blood supply.

Lymphatics: an auxiliary circulation that removes excess interstitial fluid left behind by the capillaries. It connects through lymph glands to veins above the heart.

Microvascular angina: "Syndrome X", where tiny myocardial vessels are too narrow but larger coronaries remain open.

Murmur: A sound made by the heart other than the normal heart sounds that may be associated with either normal or abnormal function.

Myocardial: pertaining to the heart muscle.

Peripheral resistance: The resistance to blood flow in either the systemic or pulmonary circuit caused by narrowing of vessels and friction of flowing blood .

Potassium (K): The predominant positively charged ion within body cells.

Regurgitation: backward leak of a valve.

Septum: partition between right and left heart chambers.

Sodium (Na): The predominant positively charged ion in the interstitial fluid outside of cells.

Stable angina: repeatable pattern of onset, usually with exercise or stress, lets up with rest or nitroglycerin.

Stenosis: blockage of a valve opposing forward motion of the blood.

Systole: the phase of the cardiac cycle when the heart muscle is contracting.

Stroke volume: amount the heart pumps out with each beat.

Tachycardia: excessively fast heart rate.

Thrombosis: blockage of a blood vessel by clot.

Transducer: A tool for sensing a body function and converting it to a readable graph.

Ventricles: right and left lower pumping chambers.

Variant angina: cardiac pain, usually during sleep, unrelated to exercise or stress.

The Author

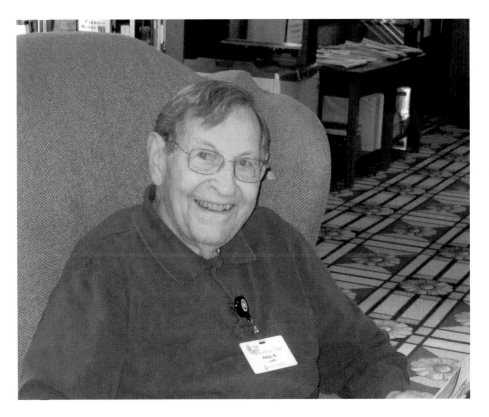

Courtesy Robert Jagoda

Dr. Lurie, age 97, at home, Woodland Pond at New Paltz, NY.

Made in the USA
Columbia, SC
14 December 2018